WHAT YOU DON'T KNOW ABOUT CANCER TREATMENT

*Awareness, Education, and Action **Are Key***

GILDA L. GONZALEZ

Paperback ISBN: 978-1-7340645-3-7

eBook ISBN: 978-1-7340645-4-4

LCCN: 2020917380

DEDICATION

I am humbly writing this dedication with sincere appreciation. If I don't mention all of those who deserve it, please forgive me. So many people have supported me in my healing journey and my life. Without you, I wouldn't be where I am now.

To God for giving me the strength I needed to stand on my feet and to get up when life knocked me down. My faith in a supreme power always holds me in times of hardship.

To cancer patients and their families: You are my main inspiration for writing this book, and I hope my story inspires you to look beyond conventional treatments to find ways to help your body become strong by utilizing its own healing systems without chemotherapy.

To my husband, Sal, the amazing man I've been blessed to have by my side, giving me unconditional love and support, for over thirty-eight years.

To my children Sal, Alfred, and Susana, who are my motivation. I am blessed by having you as my children. I have accomplished the most challenging and extraordinary things in my life, thinking of you.

To my grandson, Jovanny: I love you, Sunshine. You bring continuous joy to my life.

To my dear parents, who taught me so many values, morals, and traditions that enrich my life; and to my brothers and sisters. Thanks for being such a wonderful family.

To my amazing friends who were there with me, cheering me on to continue my healing journey. Your kind words were the inspiration to my soul. Your cards always brought me joy, and your continuous prayers most definitely were heard.

CONTENTS

INTRODUCTION

Without health, life is not life; it is only a state of languor and suffering.

—Francois Rabelais

My name is Gilda L. Gonzalez. I am the author of this book, and I am the protagonist of this story. My mission in life is to serve others by sharing my experience and the process I went through to overcome cancer. I want to share what I learned, the approaches I utilized, and the struggles I encountered during my journey to a positive outcome.

In 2013, I was diagnosed with stage III colon cancer. At that time, I had little or no knowledge of cancer treatment, and the only thing that resonated with me about cancer was untimely death. I underwent radiation and surgery, but I refused the prescribed chemotherapy.

Have you or any of your loved ones faced cancer? Do you know someone who has lost a family member or a friend to cancer? So many people struggle with questions, uncertainty, despair, pain, and frustration when facing a deadly illness like cancer.

There are so many people who have lived and died before you. You will never have a new problem; you're not going to ever have a new problem. Somebody wrote the answer down in a book somewhere.

—Will Smith

But as actor Will Smith notes, there are no problems someone else has not already explored. That thought is true for every situation, and it motivated me to look for a better way to deal with cancer.

I believe that other than death, "everything is figureoutable," as Marie Forleo, an American life coach and motivational speaker, says. With that in mind, I set out to find my options and possibilities. The more I studied valid, reliable, and authentic sources, the more astonished I was at the variety of approaches available for healing my body.

If you are reading this book, it is not a coincidence. I firmly believe there are no coincidences in this world. Something brought you here, and whatever it was, I hope you find a silver lining woven through these pages in your quest for nonintrusive healing.

All of life is peaks and valleys. Don't let the peaks get too high and the valleys too low.

—John Wooden

Wooden's words resonate with me because I was living life just by going through the motions before my diagnosis. Cancer gave me a reality check. All of a sudden, my "valley" was very low, too low. It caught me off guard and thrust me into a strange world. I had to face the deadliest illness I could imagine while being ignorant of what to do and certain that the journey would not be pleasant.

The journey taught me many lessons. Many of them were bitter, but I also must admit that the experience of healing from cancer made me a completely new person—a person who has learned to appreciate life and to realize that every day is a new day full of hope and possibilities. It taught me to become more aware of how fragile life is and made me realize how much unfinished business I had.

Do you associate the word *cancer* with death? Are you aware that there are many options available to prevent and reverse cancer?

The purpose of this book is to share what I learned and what I did to help my body regain health and rid it of cancer cells. My aim is to create awareness about cancer therapies and the one-size-fits-all approach of standard treatment, and to educate cancer patients and their families about alternative, holistic, integrative therapies available. I want to encourage you—whether you are a cancer patient or have a relative or friend who is—*not to give your power to others*, to take action and be the master of your body and your health.

I hope this book will assist you in making daily lifestyle choices that will help your body regain wellness and give you a better quality of life—for your family's sake as well as yours, because when an individual gets cancer, the entire family suffers.

I am and will continue to be a student in the quest for holistic healing, and I will continue to learn about integrative ways to keep my body and mind healthy and at their best.

FIRST THINGS FIRST

Health is a state of complete harmony of the body, mind and spirit. When one is free from physical disabilities and mental distractions, the gates of the soul open.

—B.K.S. IYENGAR

I had to go through the bitterness of a disease to find a silver lining that would help me understand how the body works and what it needs to be nourished and function optimally. Yes, I must admit that I appreciate wellness now more than ever before and more than anything money can buy in this world.

I represent a special community: cancer patients and their loved ones. This group of people suffers intensely from the moment the cancer diagnosis is announced. Most people in this community feel helpless, and although they are aware of standard cancer treatments, their experiences and their memories of others' battles with cancer are mainly negative and painful. New patients are often full of sadness and already have a mindset that they are going to die. The day of my cancer diagnosis was very painful and uncertain, with so many doubts, so much frustration and anger. I sympathize with cancer patients and want to offer hope, because cancer shouldn't be a death sentence.

I want to offer a guiding hand by providing information about what I did to conquer cancer without chemotherapy. It required taking the control of my health into my own hands. That meant being sure I was doing things right, including being consistent in implementing treatment protocols, keeping regular doctor appointments, and monitoring cancer tests.

Most of the strategies I will share are simple and free. Giving your body the essential tools it needs to heal does not have to cost a fortune. It does not have to deplete your financial resources or force you into bankruptcy.

WHY ALTERNATIVE MEDICINE?

Having balance in your body starts with identifying the stressors that eat up your wellness. The basic principles include understanding that all parts of the body are interconnected, and nothing works in isolation.

The fact that I had stage III colon cancer did not mean the problem was confined to the colon. It meant I had to identify and treat the underlying cause of the cancer. Understanding first what had put me in that situation was an important step toward finding a viable solution.

I decided to turn to "alternative" medicine because it allowed me to see my health from a wholistic perspective. Colon cancer was the symptom; it was telling me something was wrong with my body and my health in general.

According to the *Merriam-Webster Dictionary*, *alternative medicine* is "any of various systems of healing or treating disease (such as homeopathy, chiropractic, naturopathy, Ayurveda, or faith healing) that are not included in the traditional curricula taught in medical schools of the United States and Britain."

Conventional medicine is highly effective for many health conditions. But in my search for options other than chemotherapy, I decided to think outside the box and find more natural ways to give my body what it needed to heal and repair itself after battling cancer. I believe that alternative medicine's noninvasive wellness practices can make an enormous contribution to our overall health.

Unfortunately, many health insurance plans in the United States do not cover these healing methods, and some treatments, such as chiropractic, can be rather expensive—though they are relatively cheap when compared with being sick.

Holistic medicine is a form of healing that considers the whole person—mind, body, spirit, and emotions—in the quest for optimal health and wellness. According to the holistic medicine philosophy, one can achieve optimal wellness by gaining a proper balance in life. Holistic medicine practitioners believe that the whole person is made up of interdependent parts and that if one part is not working properly, all the other parts will be affected. In this way, imbalances (physical, emotional, or spiritual) in people's lives can negatively impact their overall wellness.[1]

Integrative medicine is another approach. It takes the most effective treatments from different disciplines, using standard Western medicine and complementary traditional approaches together. The result is a personalized wellness plan for your unique physical and emotional needs.

Integrative medicine is a medical specialty. This means that you can find a doctor who is board-certified in integrative medicine and trust that your treatments will be safe and proven to work. Here's what you can expect from this kind of medical care:

- A close partnership with your doctor;
- A focus on noninvasive treatments when possible;

---

1   "What Is Holistic Medicine?" WebMD, updated March 18, 2020, https://www.webmd.com/balance/guide/ what-is-holistic-medicine#1.

- Commitment to treatments based on evidence that they work;
- Consideration of everything that influences your wellness, including your home environment.[2]

WHY THIS BOOK?

I was very hesitant about writing a nonfiction book. I did not even know how to start, since I had never written a book before. I did not want to duplicate books already out there. However, as time passed, I learned of more people, including friends and close family members, being diagnosed with cancer, and it pained me to know that some were dying without having the opportunity to learn about available approaches to heal their bodies.

This book is my personal journey of beating cancer without chemo, and it could make a difference for you. I wrote it for you and other patients and their families who are in despair at hearing the word *cancer*. I lived it and know how painful not knowing where to start can be.

The first books I read about cancer were full of data and hard to understand. They had lots of numbers, statistics, and definitions that were difficult to comprehend. Although the information was valuable, at that moment, I did not have time for that. All I needed was a starting point with simple, easy-to-follow steps to give my body the extra boost it needed to regain overall wellness. I wanted clear and concise information on strategies and tools. So, this is a short book.

From the bitterness of disease, man learns the sweetness of health.

—CATALAN PROVERB

---

2   "What is Integrative Medicine?" WebMD, updated May 25, 2019, https://www.webmd.com/cancer/holistic-treatment-17/integrative-medicine.

WHAT IS CANCER?

First, some biology basics. According to CancerInstitute.org, the human body contains billions of cells. As old cells die, other cells divide to make new cells. This process happens in the body millions of times a day.

Cancers start when some cells in the body become abnormal, multiply out of control, and take over normal cells in an area of the body. These cells don't behave the same way as healthy cells do. They can grow and divide faster or live longer.[3]

As time passes, more and more abnormal cells are made, and they start to outnumber normal cells in an area of the body. They multiply out of control and form cancer.[4]

Making healthy choices can remove cancer-causing factors from your life and greatly reduce your risk of having a recurrence or dying from cancer. Awareness is the first step for change, but awareness without education and action is fruitless.

It is important to become aware of the many options to help your body heal. Then you need to continue learning, because knowledge will give you confidence in your decisions.

Some actions are very simple but powerful. Most of us know the basic principles of healthy living, but we ignore or dismiss them. As simple a habit as drinking a sufficient amount of water can help. Water hydrates your body, which helps it produce more energy. Simple exercise is another way to improve your body. Moderate exercises such as walking and stretching help your circulatory system.[5]

To understand cancer, you must first know that cancer cannot exist by itself. It exists and grows in the body. Everything we do to the body can

---

3   "What Is Cancer?" National Cancer Institute, https://www.cancer.gov/about-cancer/understanding/what-is-cancer.

4   "How Cancers Grow." Cancer Research UK. Accessed December 5, 2017. https://www.cancerresearchuk. org/about-cancer/what-is-cancer/how-cancers-grow.

5   "Benefits of Physical Activity," Centers for Disease Control and Prevention, https://www.cdc.gov/physicalactivity/basics/pa-health/index.htm.

have a good effect or a bad effect on the growth of cancer. Cancer creates its own microenvironment, and the increasingly altered body environment then feeds the cancerous cells. With a few exceptions, such as when genetics play a role (a rare occurrence), cancer is the result of a condition or group of conditions that *set up the environment* for it to grow.

For example, many colon cancers could be avoided if people paid attention to the optimum wellness of their colons. This includes drinking enough water; eating a nutritious, balanced diet; exercising; and maintaining regular bowel movements to ensure proper absorption and elimination.

Cancer does not just happen overnight, and it cannot survive in a well-nourished environment, which includes achieving a mind, body, and spirit balance. Prevention is the most desirable approach, but if you are already faced with the challenge of the illness, then a holistic approach to dealing with it must be put in place. [6]

To truly treat cancer, we have to look beyond merely killing the cancer cells. A combination of surgery, chemotherapy, and radiation was not the solution for me. I was able to understand the dynamics that surround cancer and the importance of creating an optimal environment where cancer cannot survive.

You must modify the environment that provides the optimum path for cancer's growth so that cancer finds it increasingly difficult to take root. You must empower the immune system so that it remains effective and is not a silent bystander while cancer grows. How? By starting with the nutrients you put into your body.

Avoid junk food, including food with preservatives, artificial colors, flavors, and odors. Avoid sugary drinks, refined flours, and saturated fat. It sounds complicated to understand the importance and value of each nutrient fully, but these basic recommendations can help you a ton.[7]

---

6   CDC, "Benefits of Physical Activity."

7   U. Rudrappa, Nutrition Facts blog, https://www. nutrition-and-you.com/.

Our bodies have all the tools they need to overcome most diseases. They have been doing that task from the day each of us was born. Somewhere along the way, our body's defenses got overwhelmed. Overloading the body with toxins, giving it food that's depleted of nutrients, having too much alcohol or other drugs, and emotional toxicity in the environment are among the ways an immune system can be compromised.

The body can also become overwhelmed by environmental toxins and toxic chemicals in food and body products. The reasons for getting cancer are many. That is why knowing how to restore the body's ability to defend itself is a central theme in holistic cancer medicine.

Again, cancer does not start overnight by itself.

Again, it is the result of a combination of factors, such as environmental toxins, a compromised immune system due to poor nutrition, a sedentary lifestyle, emotional toxicity, and—in rare cases—genetics.

SEEKING THE SOLUTION

I still remember the day I was diagnosed with stage III colon cancer. It was in August of 2013. That day, I felt as if my world had fallen apart. I reviewed my life from as early as I could remember in childhood to the present time, and I felt sad, thinking that my life was going to end very soon. My husband was with me, but I was so trapped in my emotions that I was not even fully aware of his presence.

I thought about the next steps I likely would have to endure—surgery, chemotherapy, and radiation. These were the only options I thought I had.

Everything seemed so pointless: my work, my many years of attending school, my attempts to do more and do better. All that mattered was that more likely than not, I would die of cancer. The most painful thing of all was that my family would have to see me die the way most cancer patients go, by slowly deteriorating. If you have been diagnosed with cancer, you probably can relate to what I am saying.

Will you have to go through the same struggles I went through? Is it true that there is no hope for cancer patients? Will you have to face the emotional pain of letting your loved ones know about your limited options for cancer treatment and slim survival probabilities? Or will you take responsibility for your wellness and become educated about different methods for helping to treat your cancer?

If I ever get cancer again, it would not be the same for me as it was when I was diagnosed with stage III colon cancer in 2013. I am now equipped with knowledge of the many alternative ways to support my body while treating cancer. I am convinced that most types of cancer are preventable and curable. I am convinced because I have already been through it.

There are hundreds, if not thousands, of documented successes using alternative therapies for cancer treatment. However, many variables play a role in the success rate. For example, the type and stage of the cancer are the two main variables that determine treatment success or failure. Does this sound discouraging? I hope not, because the success rate for cancer "remission" is on the rise.

> Half the modern drugs could well be thrown out the window, except that the birds might eat them.
>
> —Martin H. Fischer, MD

THE STANDARD TREATMENT

On the day of my diagnosis, I was referred by my gastrointestinal (GI) doctor to an oncologist and a surgeon. I was listening to the doctor's orders, but in reality, I was in a state of mind that his orders meant little to me. I agreed and followed through with his instructions and was soon scheduled for surgery and radiation.

I acquiesced to these treatments out of ignorance about existing alternative options to help my body heal and under pressure from the medical profession and from seeing my family members' sadness. My intuition, my reasoning, and what I had already learned from literature helped me to conclude that there must be better ways to heal my body, a body that was designed to heal itself but that I had neglected to listen and to protect. With that in mind, I began to read about natural, alternative, holistic approaches to help my body regain overall health and wellness, and I tried every possible method, system, and approach to give my body what it needed to heal itself.

I learned about better and less invasive ways to overcome cancer and even found several different ways to prevent it. Fortunately for me—and you—preventing illnesses and regaining wellness naturally is an option that merits consideration.

There are many practical, universal recommendations, which I will describe in later chapters, and if we followed them, we would have half the battle won.

In addition, you can take supplements under the care of a health provider and balance your body, mind, and spirit through relaxation, meditation, and other methods. These are very compelling ways of optimizing wellness. They are basic, common-sense recommendations, yet unfortunately, they are not common practices. I have to admit that it is challenging to make lifestyle changes and maintain them, but if I can do it, you can do it too.

Change is laborious, particularly when bad habits have a long history. Fortunately, habits are acquired through practice, which means that you can acquire new ones. It's tough to change when you are used to eating fast food; drinking sugary, artificial beverages; and eating flour in bread, pizza, pasta, and tortillas.

However, when you realize that your eating habits are cutting your life short, the decision to switch to healthy habits should be pretty simple. Unfortunately, few of us make the required changes until we encounter disease.

Why do most people wait until they are faced with a debilitating illness like diabetes or cancer? The answer is simple: if you do not feel the need to learn or change to a healthy lifestyle, going with the flow is effortless. Plus, many people eat "comfort food." This is not to blame or shame you; I used to do it too. It is what we learned and what we are used to, but the reality is that eventually our bodies will scream for help.

Awareness, education, and action play vital roles here. Planning is part of taking action, because once you are hungry, you will eat whatever is available. Planning your daily meals ahead of time will help you avoid those hunger bursts and binges on whatever is readily available. Fortunately, more and more people are becoming aware of the effects their food and lifestyle choices have on their bodies and their overall wellness; and it's not uncommon to see people making healthier selections when buying foods.

BECOMING AWARE

Awareness is the first step toward change. You need to become aware of the damage you are causing your body and act to prevent and/or overcome whatever illnesses you have. Awareness also includes knowing that you have options for health care. Finding these options is your responsibility, because it is unlikely that anyone will knock on your door and say, "Here are your options for regaining health." For example, there are several clinics in Mexico and other countries and some doctors in the United States who utilize specific protocols for fighting cancer and other chronic health conditions. I will cite the ones I am aware of in upcoming chapters.

> The difference between the impossible and the possible lies in a person's determination.
>
> —Tommy Lasorda

A CANCER MYTH

Tommy Lasorda's statement provided vital encouragement during my journey through the healing process. At first, though, I felt that my life was ending. I understood my limitations even as I decided to fight using all the therapies I could find.

That internal dissonance underscores a very important point: when people are diagnosed with cancer, they need a coach or mentor—a support person who fights with them and rallies them when they're feeling weak, tired, or hopeless and want to give up. I was lucky to have family members who supported me through the process.

And fortunately, although my cancer was already at stage III, the symptoms were almost unnoticeable. That gave me the strength to believe that I could still seek options beyond the standard treatment.

I knew from the bottom of my heart there were more effective methods than surgery, radiation, and chemotherapy. So I rolled up my sleeves and began to find ways to help my body regain health and overall wellness.

A myth gets in the way when discussions arise about overcoming cancer. Most of the literature from conventional medical sources states that standard treatments (surgery, radiation, and chemotherapy) are the only proven treatments for cancer. However, the success rates are discouraging for most types of cancer—a five-year survival rate is a "win."

CANCER SURVIVAL RATES

Survival rates tell you what portion of people with the same type and stage of cancer are still alive five years after they were diagnosed. These numbers can't tell you how long you will live, but they might give you a better understanding of how likely it is that your treatment will be successful. There is some speculation that survival rates are not necessarily increasing, but instead, reflect earlier identification of cancer.

According to the American Cancer Society, relative survival rates are a more accurate way to estimate the effect of cancer on survival. These rates compare people with cancer with people in the overall population. For example, if the five-year relative survival rate for a specific type and stage of cancer is 90 percent, that means that people who have that cancer are, on average, about 90 percent as likely as people who don't have that cancer to live for at least five years after being diagnosed.[8]

Remember, though, the five-year relative survival rates are estimates. Your outlook can vary based on several factors specific to you. You must learn about the survival rate for your particular type of cancer, stage, the area(s) of your body it has affected, and whether the cancer is already metastatic. (The spread of cancer cells from one tissue or organ to other parts of the body is called *metastasis*.)

Survival rates are also affected by the individual's emotional state, the availability of a moral support system, how toxic the person's body and/or mind is, and available resources.

As you read literature about cancer, you will find that these individual variables play a central role in determining survival possibilities. It is also true that once your doctor tells you how long you have to live, *and you believe it*, it most likely will play out that way. Let's not be part of that statistic.

Let's be among those courageous individuals who take wellness into their own hands and who make informed decisions about what the doctor tells them to do or not to do. Unfortunately, most of us blindly follow doctors' orders without taking everything else into account because we don't know any better. I was one of those patients, at first.

There are two days in the year that we cannot do anything: yesterday and tomorrow.

—MAHATMA GANDHI

---

8   "Stomach Cancer Survival Rates," American Cancer Society, https:// www.cancer.org/ cancer/stomach-cancer/detection-diagnosis-staging/survival-rates.html.

WHAT TO DO RIGHT NOW?

You need to decide today to take your wellness into your own hands. Act now. It is not helpful to feel regret for what did not happen or hope that something magical will occur tomorrow and you'll be cured. Although miracles do occur, most times you need to take decisive, logical, sound, and consistent actions toward your healing.

Let me repeat: you need to decide what is logical and sound based on reliable information and maintain consistency in your actions. There are no magic bullets for healing your body. Wellness, in general, works as with diet: you cannot get in shape just by eating healthy food for one day. To see sustainable results, you need to stay the course.

I am not advocating any particular protocol because I understand that every case is different. Some protocols could work for some people or certain types of cancer, and others won't. But I am convinced that there are effective methods for helping your body heal, and that we all would benefit from adopting simple health practices and making them habits. These habits will have a synergistic effect on your healing process. In my personal experience, these habits were key elements in my speedy recovery from cancer.

CHAPTER 2

WHY DID YOU GET CANCER?

Basing our happiness on our ability to control everything is futile. While we do control our choice of action, we cannot control the consequences of our choices.

—STEPHEN R. COVEY IN *FIRST THINGS FIRST*

Why do you have cancer? Why do you think cancer is so prevalent now? Why do you think approximately one in every three individuals gets cancer?

The answers to these questions could light up your life and enhance your knowledge of cancer. Answering these questions is easy and understanding the most common causes of cancer will give you a better chance of preventing cancer or reversing it.

During my research, I came to realize that small steps can make a big difference in life, even, as Stephen Covey states, "we cannot control the consequences of our choices." External forces did not control my choices related to nutrition and my emotional and spiritual state, and I had to face that reality, too.

WHY ME?

If you have cancer, you are probably asking the same questions I asked myself. You probably feel sad and hopeless. The very first thing on a cancer patient's mind after a diagnosis is usually, "Why me? Why did this happen?"

After all, *cancer* is a concept that is very distant for most of us. Unconsciously, though, most of us have it in the back of our minds, because most people have lost a friend or a family member to cancer. According to the National Cancer Institute, approximately 38.4 percent of men and women will be diagnosed with cancer at some point in their lives (based on 2013–2015 data). One in three people!

Those odds are pretty scary. They suggest that it is not a matter of *why me*; it is more a matter of *when*. Does that mean that you will be diagnosed with cancer? No. It means that you need to be aware of the high incidence of cancer; it also underlines the importance of getting educated about prevention and taking immediate action.

* * *

I vividly remember the day I was diagnosed. It was devastating to hear the words *stage III colon cancer*. I was hoping it was a nightmare. *Cancer* was a scary word and a terrifying reality that I was not ready to face. My mind was out in space, my world was ending, and in my despair, I was concerned my loved ones would suffer with me.

Since it was so painful for me, I debated internally whether to keep it to myself or to let my family know about it. But cancer is not something that you can keep to yourself for very long. Moreover, I got scared about the prospect of dying without giving my children the benefit of knowing about it ahead of time.

But let me tell you, the fear is temporary. Other feelings replace it, including uncertainty and doubt, until you eventually transition to a state of calm and peace.

This transition happened for me as I started learning about the options available to help my body regain health. When I understood that cancer was not a death sentence, all of those negative feelings began to disappear. Soon, they were replaced with hope serenity.

WERE THERE SIGNS?

Getting cancer or other health conditions never goes unpredicted. Usually by the time you are diagnosed with cancer or another chronic degenerative condition, your body has already given you signals that something is going wrong. For you to get sick with cancer, diabetes, high cholesterol, high blood pressure, etc., several factors must be present way before the diagnosis. Sometimes we just ignore them. Other times we try to diagnose ourselves or minimize symptoms because we are afraid of finding out the truth.

If you have cancer, you may have gotten it because your body was overloaded with toxins, and that compromised your immune system. Those toxins could be the result of poor nutritional habits; environmental factors; unhealthy ingredients in the products you put on your body, including lotions, creams, shampoo, and makeup; and/or emotional wounds from previous life experiences. Additional risk factors that increase the chances of getting cancer are physiological. They include, for example, chronic health conditions like diabetes, high cholesterol, and obesity. Your immune system is the first line of defense. It must be working properly to be able to identify malignant cells and destroy them before they grow and spread.

My body had been telling me something was wrong. I felt tired. I was losing weight despite the fact that I was not doing anything intentionally to shed pounds. I had a history of constipation to which I was not giving proper attention, and I was noticing some bloody spots in the stool. I had dismissed those signals. However, once I understood that I was the only person responsible for what was going wrong with my body, I decided to make steady changes to my unhealthy habits.

I took simple steps, like developing healthier eating habits. I began to eat lots of vegetables and fruits and made sure that food portions were proportionally distributed to include enough protein, carbohydrates, and fiber.

Be careful of making hurried, uneducated, or poorly informed decisions. Cancer does not develop overnight. Because of that, in my opinion, there is no need for you to rush into an invasive treatment. Current cancer treatments could change your life forever. If cancer has been in your body for months or years before diagnosis, another month shouldn't kill you. The decision is always yours.

Take the time to get a second opinion, because some research indicates that many cancer diagnoses are false positives. That could mean that some patients have received or are receiving cancer treatment by mistake.[9] In his book *The Truth About Cancer*, Ty Bollinger explains the that 99 percent of all mammogram referrals are false positives. Citing a paper published in *The Lancet*, he maintains that the PSA test for prostate cancer yields similar poor results. "High levels of PSA can mean many other things besides cancer, yet nearly every man who scores high on the test is urged to undergo a prostate biopsy, an extremely invasive procedure that, again, like mammograms for women, can lead to the spread of cancer cells from the site of a possible tumor to the rest of the body."[10] You have the power to decide what is done to your body. Become informed.

---

9   Ty Bollinger, *The Truth About Cancer* (Carlsbad, California; Hay House, 2018), p. 123–124.

10   *The Truth About Cancer*, p. 123–124.

DECISIONS MATTER

It is believed that the main pillars of wellness are nutrition, maintaining a healthy environment, and achieving a state of emotional well-being. Therefore, the diet and lifestyle decisions you've made up to this point have all affected your health.

They had certainly affected mine. My lifestyle had opened the door to sickness. For example, before cancer, I consumed a diet high in carbohydrates, including tortillas, pasta, white rice, and the like, which lack nutritional value. For me, with my long history of suffering from constipation, a more appropriate diet is one high in fiber from foods such as apples, lentils, beans, avocados, broccoli, and cauliflower—in general, a plant-based diet.

It is believed that most cancers are caused by poor diet and lifestyle choices, emotional distress, and environmental factors, and I believe that these factors are the root of many other chronic health conditions as well. So, if the problem has already been identified, the solution should be simple: awareness, education, and action. The more you can reduce your body's toxic load, the better your odds are of preventing or healing cancer.

I am living proof that it can be done. Learning about my body's ability to repair itself was amazing because it gave me the power to utilize the tools needed to support it in this endeavor.

Among the changes I made was consuming nutrition-dense food, including vegetables, legumes, and some fruit. I eliminated sugary drinks and instead drank water and coconut water, which is credited with many health benefits. I eliminated meat from my diet while I was doing the core treatment, although eventually I incorporated free-range, hormone- and antibiotic-free meat in small amounts. I also started taking supplements, including multivitamins and minerals such as a magnesium, zinc, manganese, iodine, and selenium. Vitamin D3 was also part of my anti-cancer protocol. I became very mindful and intentional of what I ate and did each and every day. Supporting my body to function properly became my new "normal."

Unfortunately, even though most of us know what to do, few of us do it. For example, most of us know how important it is to drink lots of water instead of sugary drinks, but we do not do it. We know how important it is to exercise and eat healthy food, but we do not do it.

You could read a hundred books. You could listen to social media documentaries and go to all the seminars and workshops in the world. But if you do not take consistent action toward sustainable results, then your knowledge won't help.

We all need to understand that the incidence of cancer among us is very high. But this incidence is not set in stone. The statistic is an average. So, do not become one of the people diagnosed with cancer.

How? By making progressive and sustainable changes to decrease your risk of getting cancer. It is not just about changing your diet; it is about changing your lifestyle to one that makes it almost impossible for cancer cells to grow. If you already have cancer, the answer to a better outcome is in your hands now.

People often get inspired when reading books or listening to motivational speakers, but the challenging part is to stay the course. And remember, if making a radical change is difficult for you, that is absolutely normal. Start with baby steps.

If you regress, start again. And again. Start as many times as you need to until it becomes a habit. Changes are more difficult at the beginning and become easier with time. Do not give up. You'll start to see and feel the difference in your body's overall wellness. I will end this section with the following quote, which resonates very strongly with me. I hope it does with you too.

Life is like riding a bicycle. To keep your balance, you must keep moving.

—ALBERT EINSTEIN

EDUCATE YOURSELF

A few years ago, I read that there is almost nothing in this world that someone hasn't already written about, and there are different types of experts. There are those who have lived through an experience, learned along the way, and succeeded. The other type of expert is the research expert.

If you have been diagnosed with cancer, commit to getting educated. There are hundreds of well-researched books about helping your body regain wellness. There are no excuses for ignorance now.

When people are diagnosed with this dreaded disease, they often feel paralyzed, and that makes it more difficult to do anything concrete about it. That's why it is imperative for cancer patients to have a person whom they trust to support them during the treatment process.

If you are the family member or a friend of a cancer patient, to be able to help that patient you need to understand some basics about cancer—where it comes from, how it develops, what type of cancer it is, the stage, etc. More importantly, you need to know about alternative, holistic approaches for that specific situation. You need to become a research expert.

Fighting cancer is not an easy task. It is a process that requires discipline. In most cases, it requires multiple approaches. Throughout this book, I will remind you that unless it is a real emergency, do not rush into the standard treatment of radiation, surgery, and/or chemotherapy.

Why would you throw a bomb into your garage to kill a mouse, if you can kill the mouse without destroying your garage?

There are better ways to do almost everything, and cancer treatment is no exception. At the time of my diagnosis, I was like most of you. I was ignorant about where to start as far as integrative or alternative medicine is concerned. I was ignorant about the dozens, if not hundreds, of alternative methods there are to heal most cancers.

Rushing into radiation and surgery was a big mistake for me. The more I became educated about cancer, the more I understood what my body went through during the standard treatment. If I ever get cancer again, I will never accept the conventional treatment, because the side effects I experienced from radiation and surgery were devastating and had lifelong consequences.

My point is that there is no need to rush into the standard treatment. You need to get all the facts in your hands first, including treatment options, length of treatment, the percentage of success, and alternative ways to heal. Even if you decide to go with the traditional approach to treat cancer, my advice is to do it based on facts, so you will not regret it when it is too late to change course.

Learning is effortless today, particularly if you have access to the internet. A word of caution, though: make sure that the information comes from trusted and reliable sources.

I soon understood the harmful elements that were impacting my wellness, and I knew that I had to make big changes. I knew that even if I was able to make it through the standard treatment, the prognosis might not be favorable because my overall wellness was not optimal. At the time, my lifestyle did not favor the healing process.

When I began to research why I had cancer, I was astonished to learn how sugar damages your immune system and how cancer sustains itself mainly on sugar. Thinking back, I recalled the dozens of TV commercials I'd seen that targeted children and families in general with the message: consume sugary products. I thought about the many food items high in sugar I used to have in my home—soft drinks, cereal, cookies, pastries, etc. Interestingly, when I completed my radiation therapy, I was given two tickets for free ice cream! I had similar experiences in the hospitals where I had surgery. This is hilarious! If cancer cells feed on sugar, why would a cancer institution provide patients with sugar as a reward for completing a cancer treatment?

In *Beating Cancer with Nutrition*, Dr. Patrick Quillin writes, "Sugar is cancer's favorite food. There are at least five reasons that cancer and sugar are best friends. Cancer cells love sugar! That is why refined carbohydrates like white sugar, white flour, high fructose corn syrup (HFCS) and soft drinks are extremely dangerous for anyone trying to prevent or reverse cancer. Sugar essentially feeds tumors and encourages cancer growth. Cancer cells uptake sugar at ten to twelve times the rate of healthy cells. In fact, that is the basis of PET (positron emission tomography) scans—one of the most accurate tools for detecting cancer growth. PET scans use radioactively labeled glucose to identify sugar-hungry tumor cells. When patients drink the sugary water before the scan, it gets preferentially taken up into the cancer cells and they light up! The 1931 Nobel laureate in medicine, German Otto Warburg, Ph.D., discovered that cancer cells have a fundamentally different energy metabolism compared to healthy cells. He found that malignant tumors exhibit increased glycolysis—a process whereby glucose is used as fuel by cancer—as compared with normal cells."[11]

It is unbelievable how this simple but important concept is not shared with cancer patients. Cancer patients are directed to follow doctors' orders with minimal information or explanation and few recommendations for food selection. If cancer cells consume over ten times more sugar than normal cells, it is extremely wise to eliminate sugar intake, particularly the added sugar in processed foods and sugary drinks.

Should you eliminate sugar from your diet completely? No, because normal cells also need sugar, but the amount they need is much less. You get sugar from fruits and some vegetables. Low-glycemic fruits are recommended when getting treated for cancer. It is important to get educated on which fruits and vegetables are recommended for your type of cancer. Obtaining valid and reliable information from nutritionists, credible websites, or by hiring a coach would be the safest way when deciding what to eat and what not to eat.

I am not blaming well-intentioned doctors. They are prescribing the

---

11   Patrick Quillin, *Beating Cancer with Nutrition* (Carlsbad, California, 2005).

treatment they believe will work for their patients; after all, it is what they learned in medical school. Instead of pointing fingers, which is a waste of time for a cancer patient trying to get well, educate yourself. Be mindful of what you are getting into, take your wellness into your own hands, and do not allow others to decide for you.

STRESS, CANCER, AND YOUR IMMUNE SYSTEM

Chronic stress is considered one of the main factors in getting cancer. It's the one thing that can outweigh everything else you do. It is difficult to identify daily stressors, such as getting through traffic and dropping children off at school while trying to get to work on time. That kind of stress is different from toxic stress.

Many of us live life by just going through the motions and experience chronic stress from many angles of our lives, including family, personal, and work-related stress. No matter what you do, if your level of chronic stress is always high, it could be compromising your immune system.

The relationship between stress and cancer and other diseases is complex. Research studies have demonstrated that chronic or long-term stress dramatically suppresses the immune system.

The National Center for Biotechnology Information's (NCBI) meta-analysis of three hundred articles revealed that "chronic stressors were associated with suppression of both cellular and humoral measures. Effects of event sequences varied according to the kind of event (trauma vs. loss)."[12]

Understanding the immune system and its relationship with chronic illnesses is more complicated than you may think. It is my personal opinion based on my own experience and literature review that chronic stress should be addressed as part of the cancer treatment to maximize its effectiveness.

---

12   Suzanne C Segerstrom and Gregory E Miller, "Psychological stress and the human immune system: a meta-analytic study of 30 years of inquiry," *Psychological Bulletin* vol. 130,4 (2004): 601-30. doi:10.1037/0033-2909.130.4.601, abstract.

It is essential to identify your level of stress and do something about it. In *Healing the Addicted Brain*, author Harold C. Urschel III, MD, stresses the importance of utilizing relaxation techniques to help keep your stress level low. He writes, "Practicing relaxation on a regular basis is the best way to lower your anxiety levels and give your body and mind a 'vacation' from stress."[13]

One of my favorite relaxation techniques is doing four cycles of proper deep breathing four times a day. It supplies the brain with oxygen, so I think more clearly. It also improves circulation and digestion. Isn't that enough for you to want to get into the habit and make deep breathing part of your ongoing regimen? You do not have to complicate your life to do deep breathing. You can do it while driving, standing, walking, or lying down, so there are no excuses not to benefit from this great exercise.

Another strategy to help you relax is journaling. This relaxation method has been used in different fields, including psychology. The simple practice of regular journaling releases tension from your body, which could improve your sleep rhythm and keep you from waking up in the middle of the night.

Buy a journal or notebook and try it for one month. Every night before going to bed, write down whatever happened during the day, including any concerns you may have, and list upcoming commitments. Once you have put these thoughts down on paper, you do not have to worry about them as much as when you try to hold them in your head.

As you can see, cancer is caused by many factors. As such, you need multiple approaches to kill cancer cells.

---

13   Harold C. Urschel III, MD, *Healing the Addicted Brain*: the Revolutionary Science-Based Alcoholism and Addiction Recovery Program. (Naperville, Illinois: Sourcebooks, 2009) p. 138.

TAKE CONTROL

Everything in life happens for a reason. Most of the time, the reason is clear. The decisions you have made in the past impact your reality today, and whatever you do today will affect your life tomorrow.

Cancer is not a death sentence. Do not allow fear to take control of you, and do not allow others to make decisions for you. Be the master of your wellness and learn and apply basic health principles.

Ask for support from family members and friends. You'll need them to be at your side during the healing journey, as it is difficult to do it alone. And if you have a family member or friend who is going through cancer and you could be the person to support him or her, do it. Believe me, it is absolutely necessary.

If some of the reasons for getting cancer involve diet, lifestyle, environment, and/or stress, you need to know which of these conditions apply most to you. As you can see, all of the reasons mentioned above are of common knowledge to most of us. What matters is what you do with that knowledge. Remember: *awareness, education, and action.*

In the next chapter, we will discuss diagnosis, screening, and tests available for cancer.

CHAPTER 3

THE DIAGNOSIS

Getting diagnosed with cancer is a pretty terrifying experience for everyone. It is especially worrisome if you are not aware of what it means to have cancer. Most people associate the word *cancer* with death. What to do then? What do you need to know about cancer?

In this book, I will explain it in very elementary terms because, when you are diagnosed with cancer, you are most likely not interested in all the research behind it—at least not at that point in time. Basic, simple-to-understand information is most important at that moment. Once you get on the right track, I encourage you to continue learning about cancer so you can be better equipped for the journey that is ahead of you. The more you know about cancer—how it starts, develops, and spreads, and most importantly, how can it be prevented and even reversed—the better equipped you will be to deal with it.

HOW CANCER GROWS

Most trusted sources, such as the Cancer Treatment Center of America, define cancer as the uncontrolled growth of abnormal cells in the body. Cancer develops when the body's normal control mechanism stops working. Old cells do not die but instead grow out of control, forming new, abnormal cells. These extra cells may build a mass of tissue, called a tumor, although some cancers, such as leukemia, do not develop tumors.[14]

The National Cancer Institute explains it like this:

Cancer is the name given to a collection of related diseases. In all types of cancer, some of the body's cells begin to divide without stopping and spread into surrounding tissues. Cancer can start almost anywhere in the human body, which is made up of trillions of cells. Normally, human cells grow and divide to form new cells as the body needs them. When cells grow old or become damaged, they die, and new cells take their place. When cancer develops, however, this orderly process breaks down. As cells become more and more abnormal, old or damaged cells survive when they should die, and new cells form when they are not needed. These extra cells can divide without stopping and may form growths called tumors.[15]

The American Cancer Society explains it in this way:

Cancer can start any place in the body. It starts when cells grow out of control and crowd out healthy cells. This makes it hard for the body to work the way it should.

Many cancers can be treated. In fact, more people than ever before

---

14   "What is cancer?" Cancer Treatment Centers of America, https://www.cancercenter.com/what-is-cancer.

15   "What Is Cancer?" National Cancer Institute, https://www.cancer.gov/about-cancer/understanding/what-is-cancer.

live full lives after cancer treatment.[16]

Some cancer cells stay within the body tissue in which they have developed—for example, the lining of the colon or the bladder. This type of cancer is called *superficial cancer growth* or *carcinoma in situ*. The cancer cells grow and divide to create more cells, and eventually form a tumor. Organs have membranes that keeps the cells of that tissue inside.

Cancer cells can break through this membrane, and if that happens, the cancer is said to be *invasive*. One of the things that makes cancer cells different from normal cells is that they can move about more easily. So, it seems likely that one of the ways that cancers spread through nearby tissues is by the cells directly moving.

Malignant tumors are made up of cancer cells. They usually grow faster than benign tumors, spread into surrounding tissues, and cause damage. They may spread to other parts of the body via the bloodstream or through the lymph system to form secondary tumors. This is called *metastasis*.

A LITTLE BIT OF CONTEXT

The reasons for getting cancer vary. For example, carcinogens are known to cause it. Carcinogens are substances found in many products, including chemicals in tobacco smoke and chemicals in body lotions, shampoos, and cosmetic products. Many agents, including radiation, chemicals, and viruses, have been found to induce cancer in both experimental animals and humans. Solar ultraviolet radiation is also known to cause cancer. A lot of people believe that genetics is the primary cause of cancer; however, that has yet to be proven for all cases.[17]

I came to realize that ignorance could cost me my life. Ignorance of how my body was telling me that it needed attention; ignorance about

---

16   "What Is Cancer?" American Cancer Society, https://www.cancer.org/cancer/cancer-basics/what-is-cancer.html.

17   "Cancer Epigenetics," Cancer Quest, https://www.cancerquest.org/cancer-biology/cancer-epigenetics

the importance of taking my wellness into my own hands; and ignorance about seeking second and third opinions—or as many as needed—before undergoing procedures, which, in my case, changed my life forever.

I went through two surgeries. The initial one was to remove a section of the colon where the tumor had formed. During this procedure, I had an ileostomy, a procedure in which a piece of the ileum is diverted to an artificial opening in the abdominal wall. This procedure was done to let the colon rest and recover, and in my case, because radiation therapy had damaged the colon surrounding the tumor.

The second surgery was to remove the ileostomy and reconnect the sections of colon. Both of these surgeries tremendously stressed my body. A surgery is always a serious procedure, and when it involves a main body organ, it is even more traumatic. Going through radiation was also detrimental to my body, physically and emotionally. I got an ileostomy after surgery because of the negative effects of radiation therapy. I would probably not have needed an ileostomy if I had not received radiation.

Having an ileostomy is a life-changing process. Although the literature indicates that most people can handle it with minor trouble, that was not the case for me. I had to stay home or close to home during the four months I had it. My skin rejected it, and having it glued to my stomach was more than a challenge. I also blame that surgery for the damage to one of my kidneys, as a urinary blockage caused one kidney to stop working.

I tend to save important documents for reference and so I was able to compare lab work and other screenings from before and after the surgery. I noticed out-of-range test results for kidney function. But unfortunately, it was already too late.

I brought this concern to the attention of my primary doctor, who recommended that I drink more water. That advice would be appropriate for most people, but what I really needed was individualized attention and consideration of the fact that I had just gone through cancer treatment, including colon surgery. One year after surgery, this recommendation of drinking more water was not making any improvements in my lab work, so I decided to see a kidney doctor. This specialist discovered that my kidney was only working at 3 percent, and there was nothing to be done about it. Long story short, according to my nephrologist, symptoms such as extreme fatigue, high blood pressure, low energy, and tiredness were likely caused by my kidney shutting down due to the urinary blockage during the colon surgery.

I was ignorant and trusted in doctors' "expertise." I did not question simple and evident situations that indicated something was wrong with my body.

I don't need to go into too much detail about this tremendous kidney tragedy, but the reality is that one of my kidneys was damaged during the cancer treatment, and none of the medical experts noticed that early enough to save it. My ignorance contributed to this, because I trusted the experts to look after my health when the reality was that their attention was superficial. I was just one of many on their daily patient lists.

But for you, it could mean the difference between being well and being ill. It is almost impossible for you to know about every aspect of how your body functions, but a basic understanding and listening to your body could save you a lot of headaches and frustrations.

A year before my diagnosis in 2013, I had seen the gastrointestinal (GI) doctor, who had prescribed a colonoscopy. The results indicated that I had hemorrhoids. I received treatment for hemorrhoids even though I wasn't experiencing any hemorrhoid symptoms, such as pain, discomfort, or itching. I received this treatment with instructions to get another colonoscopy in five years. However, a year later, I went to see another GI doctor because I was not comfortable with the initial diagnosis of hemorrhoids.

This time, the GI doctor requested a sigmoidoscopy. The test showed that I had stage III colon cancer. He told me I needed immediate surgery, and I was instructed to consult an oncologist as well. I sought a second opinion to confirm the diagnosis. This second doctor requested a colonoscopy with an ultrasound.

After confirming the cancer diagnosis, his recommendations were surgery, radiation, and chemotherapy. I followed through with radiation and then surgery. I did it based on fear, on a lack of education about integrative/holistic less-invasive treatments, and because I did not take time to look for other recommendations. I thought I was running out of time, and I panicked.

THE DOCTORS' RECOMMENDATIONS

Stage III colon cancer is a pretty worrisome diagnosis. I had radiation and surgery as per the recommendations of the surgeon and the oncologist. However, I refused chemotherapy. Chemotherapy in pill form was prescribed, but I didn't want to undergo chemo. I had vivid images of people suffering during that treatment. When I went to see the oncologist halfway through the radiation treatment, he got upset with me because I had not followed his orders. He had told me to take chemotherapy pills concurrently with the radiation therapy.

But I had already learned about the awful side effects of chemotherapy, including but not limited to nausea, vomiting, hair loss, and appetite loss. I had also learned that most types of chemo do not discriminate between healthy and cancer cells but instead kill cells indiscriminately. So, I decided to say no to chemotherapy. I continued with the radiation treatment, and a couple of months after I finished it, I underwent surgery—a surgery that was long and meticulous. Recuperation was slow and painful; and I had to stay in the hospital for almost a week. After surgery, I went back to see the oncologist, as the protocol indicated.

He seemed upset again because I had not followed through with the prescribed chemotherapy pills. This time, he prescribed chemotherapy through injection. He told me to make an appointment with the front desk to have a catheter implanted to receive chemotherapy via injection.

At that point, over six months after the cancer diagnosis, I had acquired enough knowledge to make a more informed decision, and I didn't want my body to go through a poisonous procedure. I left the office and did not go back.

I am appreciative of conventional medicine because most likely, the doctors prescribed what they thought was the best treatment for me. From the doctor's perspective, most likely chemotherapy was prescribed to kill any remaining cancer cells that were not eliminated during the radiation and surgery. But I decided to go with the holistic approach and utilized resources and protocols promising to kill cancer cells without damaging my body. My goal was to strengthen my immune system, which was ultimately responsible for killing cancer/malignant cells.

I have to admit that the devastating side effects of chemo that I had read about terrified me. During my frequent visits to doctors' offices and clinics, it was heartbreaking to see evidence of the negative impact of chemotherapy in the general appearance of other patients.

In addition, it was extremely painful to imagine my family suffering along with me if I decided to accept chemotherapy as one of the treatment options. I also learned that chemotherapy could *cause* cancer because it is carcinogenic by its very nature. In *The Truth About Cancer*, Ty Bollinger writes, "Chemotherapy actually strengthens cancer cells by turning them into stem cells which are 'master' cells from which other cells are birthed."[18] Besides being so harmful for the human body, chemotherapies have a very low success rate, offering "roughly 2 percent chance of success to most cancer patients who receive them. The results of a 14-year study published in the *Journal of Clinical Oncology* in 2004 revealed that among 154,971 cancer patients from both Australia and the United States representing 22 different types of cancer, a mere 2.3 percent and 2.1 percent, respectively,

---

18   *The Truth About Cancer*, p. 75.

survived for longer than five years after undergoing chemotherapy."[19]

Chemotherapy has also long-lasting side effects. According to the Mayo Clinic, "Chemotherapy drugs can also cause side effects that don't become evident until months or years after treatment. Late side effects vary depending on the chemotherapy drug but can include: damage to lung tissue, heart problems, infertility, kidney problems, nerve damage (peripheral neuropathy), and risk of a second cancer."[20]

For those reasons, I understood that chemotherapy was going to do more harm than good, so I refused to accept it as part of my treatment. Now I know that was the best decision I could have made.

With faith in God and His infinite power and with a strong desire to live, I was able to go through the process of healing cancer without chemotherapy. I wanted to live because I love life and I felt that my mission in life was not over yet.

Not only I was afraid of chemotherapy treatment because of the side effects, but something deep in my heart prevented me from accepting it. The side effects of chemotherapy are devastating, and although it is most likely true that some types of chemotherapy are effective on certain types of cancer, it is also true that chemotherapy does not distinguish between good and bad cells. It kills them indiscriminately, leaving your body susceptible to other infections and devastating side effects.

One of the first books I read about healing cancer was *Beating Cancer with Nutrition* by Dr. Patrick Quillin. This book helped me to see a silver lining in my darkness. After reading and rereading it, I came to realize that there was hope for me. That is why I urge you to create your own awareness and take action. Doing the research will give you the information you need to heal your body. Remember, if you keep doing what you are doing, you will keep getting what you are getting.

____

19   *The Truth About Cancer*, p. 78.

20   "Chemotherapy," Mayo Clinic, accessed July 21, 2020, https://www.mayoclinic.org/tests-procedures/chemotherapy/about/pac-20385033.

There are several excellent books on nutrition. Some focus on nutrition in general; others stress the importance of particular diets like the ketogenic method, Gerson therapy, paleo, or the raw food diet. Other books focus on a person's blood type to suggest the kind of food that is suitable for them. Your best bet is to listen to your gut and trust your instincts and a good healthcare practitioner.

PERSPECTIVE MATTERS

According to the literature, most cancers are present for months or years prior to diagnosis. During those years, most of us are living normal lives. However, as soon as you get the cancer diagnosis, your perspective changes. Your appearance even seems different than it did just the day before the diagnosis.

When we strongly believe that something we've been told is true, that situation often comes to pass. That's why when an oncologist tells cancer patients that they have X amount of time to live, the patients usually hit that mark and then die.

But I vividly remember a passage in *Good to Great* by Jim Collins. He writes about Darwin Smith, who was diagnosed with nose and throat cancer. Doctors predicted that he had less than a year to live. But Smith had the strength to beat the odds. He lived for *twenty-five* more years.

The point is that your emotional state has a lot to do with how you deal with this disease. It is your responsibility to accept or reject the death sentence. No human being, not even a doctor, has the right to tell you how long you have left to live or what to do about it.

Soon after I became educated about cancer and the vast number of ways to treat it without chemotherapy, my perspective about it entirely changed. I knew there were less invasive and more effective ways to treat cancer. I did not accept the prognosis that my life would be cut short. I decided to take control of my health and wellness instead of handing total control to the doctors.

Again, become aware of the options you have, educate yourself about ways help your body regain wellness, and take action.

Brendon Burchard, an author and personal development trainer, has a saying that resonates with me: "Common sense is not always common practice." This is true for many aspects of your life. You could have all the knowledge in this world, but if you do not act on it, that knowledge is useless.

It is believed that it takes about twenty-one days to change a habit. Action—changing a habit—can be difficult at first, so start slow. Every step counts. For example, if you do not exercise at all, start walking for ten to twenty minutes a day at least three days a week.

If you have a habit of watching TV or spending a lot of time in other unproductive activities, changing it for a more rewarding habit, such as exercising, would bring you many benefits. You would be more flexible, for example, and your digestive system would work better.

If you are used to drinking sugary beverages, start by reducing the number of those drinks you consume each day and instead drink water. You will soon start noticing the results, and those results will motivate you to continue.

Now that I think back, it's very satisfying that I was able to turn weakness, despair, pain, and frustration into strength and make a stand for my health. At the time of this writing, it's been six years since my surgery, and I remain healthier than ever. Having cancer was a turning point in my life. It reminded me of how fragile life can be and how important it is to give attention to what is most valuable. It taught me to be more aware and mindful of what I do and how I do it.

Cancer was also a lesson in how to appreciate life more. It was not that I wanted to have cancer; the day I found out about it was a very painful episode in my life. However, if it weren't for cancer, I would not be where I am now, trying to help others and living a meaningful, grateful life. That challenge gave me the opportunity to learn how important it is to take care of our bodies and how important it is to create awareness about health and healthy lifestyles.

GENES OR LIFESTYLE?

I will detour a little bit here to give parents a message. As parents and caregivers, we have the responsibility to cultivate good eating habits in our children, because those habits will carry. We have all heard the statement, "You are what you eat."

Most of our eating habits come from childhood. It's little wonder members of the same family often get the same illnesses.

Lifestyles are learned and are usually passed on from generation to generation. Family members from the same household often eat the same unhealthy foods, have the same poor exercising habits, share the same toxic emotional environment, and more. It's certain that some of these factors contribute to the development of their cancers. Research demonstrates that relatively few cancers (less than 10 percent) are due to genetics. According to the authors of *The China Study*, a book about the China Project, which examined the connection between diet and disease in 6,500 men and women, "the proportion of colon cancer cases attributed to known inherited genes is only about to 1-3 percent."[21]

When I was diagnosed with cancer, I came to realize that my life consisted of going through the motions, doing the same things every day. I followed the same routines at work, at home, and with family and friends. I took it for granted that my body would function well, but suddenly, there I was, diagnosed with stage III colon cancer. I reflected on my almost fifty years and was shocked by how fast they had gone by. At that point, I realized that I had been living my life in autopilot mode. I was not living in the moment. I was either living in the past and regretting what I had or hadn't done or living in the future, worrying about events

---

21   T. Colin Campbell, PhD; and Thomas Campbell, MD; *The China Study* (Dallas: Ben-Bella Books, 2016), p. 176.

that perhaps would never happen.

The cancer diagnosis and its healing journey gave me the opportunity to see life from another perspective. I have learned to appreciate every moment in my life, and I am more aware of how important it is to balance work, personal life, professional life, and most importantly, family life. I am still in one piece and hoping to serve you by sharing my struggles and successes through cancer—one of the scariest illnesses in modern society.

Many of you have probably heard that cancer is silent. That is most likely true in the majority of cases. The important thing is to avoid opening the door for cancer to begin in your body. Prevention is so important. Before I get into screening and tests for cancer, let me mention some actions you can take to prevent almost any disease.

1. Get enough rest. Take time during the day to rest your body and mind.

2. Eat nutritious food. Nutritious food means real food, whole food. Visit the produce section of the supermarket instead of the aisles where you would find mostly manmade food. Every food item that comes in a box has been processed with preservatives and other additives to extend shelf life for months or even years. Make it a habit to eat lots of fruits and vegetables each and every day. If you have children, this is a great investment in their health. As you model healthy eating habits, you are teaching them to eat healthier when they grow up. Children learn more by example than by hearing directives from parents.

3. Drink clean water.

I will expand on all of those topics in later chapters. I know you are probably thinking it's easier said than done, but these actions eventually become habits in your daily life.

HOW IS CANCER DIAGNOSED?

Cancer is known as the silent killer because often symptoms are not present until the later stages. In my case, cancer was discovered at stage III and would probably have gone unnoticed for a few more years if I hadn't doubted the initial diagnosis of hemorrhoids and sought a second opinion.

I had had a colonoscopy the previous year with a normal result. One would think that once you have had a colonoscopy, you are safe and do not have to worry about it for the next five to ten years.

Not in my case. I was advised by my GI doctor to repeat the colonoscopy in five years. But waiting that long could have been fatal for me.

What next? Well, let's start by not freaking out about unnecessary screenings and tests.

You need to become educated before you get into a screening frenzy. You need to analyze your situation and decide whether a certain screening will be helpful to *you*. For example, if you are a woman and regularly get pap smears and the results come back normal, there is no need for you to get a vaginal ultrasound.

If a breast thermography result is normal, most likely you do not need a mammogram. The same applies to other screenings, such as those for the prostate-specific antigen (PSA) test and tumor markers.

Having said that, if the screening results are normal but you do not feel well, or you are in doubt about the result—as in my case—do a follow-up as soon as possible for peace of mind. Remember, there is usually a margin for false positive and false negative results. It is important to listen to your body; no one knows your body better than you do.

There are specific blood tests for different cancers. Measuring the human chorionic gonadotropin (HCG) hormones in nonpregnant women or men may reveal cancers in the uterus or testes, respectively. The Prostate Health Index (PHI) measures the level of prostate-specific antigen several ways; the TK1 enzyme test; and tests like the ONCOblot®, which claims to detect cancer when it's just the size of a pinhead in the body. That's true prevention.

If you can stay on top of your wellness by monitoring your health rather than just guessing whether you're moving in the right direction, there is no reason to fear cancer.

According to the American Cancer Society, the following are common cancer screenings.

FOR COLON CANCER:

- Stool-based tests such as the yearly fecal immunochemical test (FIT), the yearly guaiac-based fecal occult blood test (gFOBT), and the multitargeted stool DNA test (MT-sDNA) every three years.
- Visual (structural) exams of the colon and rectum, such as the colonoscopy, every ten years; the CT colonography (virtual colonoscopy) every five years; and the flexible sigmoidoscopy every five years

FOR ENDOMETRIAL CANCER:

The American Cancer Society recommends that at menopause, all women should be told about the risks and symptoms of endometrial cancer. Watch for symptoms, such as unusual spotting or bleeding not related to menstrual periods, and report these to a health-care provider. The Pap test is good at finding cancer of the cervix, but it's not a test for endometrial cancer.

FOR CERVICAL CANCER:

Cervical cancer can affect any woman who is or has been sexually active. It occurs in women who have had the human papilloma virus (HPV). This virus is passed on during sex. Cervical cancer is also more likely in women who smoke, have HIV or AIDS, have poor nutrition, and who do not get regular Pap tests.

Cervical cancer testing should start at age twenty-one. Women between ages twenty-one and twenty-nine should have a Pap test done every three years. There's also a test called the HPV test. HPV testing should not be used in this age group unless it's needed after an abnormal Pap test result.

Women between the ages of thirty and sixty-five should have a Pap test plus an HPV test (called "co-testing") done every five years. This is the preferred approach, but it's OK to have a Pap test alone every three years.

Women over age sixty-five who have had regular cervical cancer testing in the past ten years with normal results should not be tested for cervical cancer. Once testing is stopped, it should not be started again. Women with a history of cervical precancer should continue to be tested for at least twenty years after that diagnosis, even if testing continues past age sixty-five.

A woman who has had a total hysterectomy (removal of her uterus and her cervix) for reasons not related to cervical cancer and who has no history of cervical cancer or serious precancer need not be tested.

A woman who has been vaccinated against HPV should still follow the screening procedure.

FOR PROSTATE CANCER:

Screenings for men may include a digital rectal exam (DRE) and possibly a prostate-specific antigen (PSA) blood test.

FOR TESTICULAR CANCER:

This uncommon cancer develops in a man's testicles, the reproductive glands that produce sperm. Most cases occur between the ages of twenty and fifty-four. The American Cancer Society recommends that all men have a testicular exam when they see a doctor for a routine physical. Men at higher risk (a family history or an undescended testicle) should talk with a doctor about additional screening. Some doctors advise regular self-exams—gently feeling for hard lumps, smooth bumps, or changes in the size or shape of the testes.

FOR BREAST CANCER:

On its website, the American Cancer Society lists the mammogram, ultrasound imaging, the breast MRI, and molecular breast imaging (MBI) as among the cancer screens that your doctor can order and cites new imaging tests that are being developed.[22] Be aware, though, that most doctors will order mammography to screen for breast cancer instead of an ultrasound, which is less invasive, less costly, and more precise.

In the 2015 documentary *The Truth about Cancer: A Global Quest*, Ty Bollinger and some experts promoted the use of different technologies to detect cancer, including thermography, a digital infrared thermographic imaging technique, as a safer way to screen for breast cancer than mammograms.

Thermography reads the heat of physiological changes that are going on in the body and is said to detect cancer when it's the size of a pinhead—way before it's a lump or a bump that can be detected on an X-ray or mammogram. Also, there is no ionizing radiation in thermography, so it can be done on a one-time basis or as often as one wants.

All cancers go through a process called neoangiogenesis, which is new blood vessel growth. Cancers grow faster than healthy tissue around them. They have to have their own discreet blood supply when they are just a couple of years old, and thermography can pick them up just as they are getting that new blood vessel supply and the blood vessels are warm.

Mammography is about 67 percent accurate at finding cancers when they are pea size, and since most breast cancers are slow growing, by the time they are detected, they are already eight years old.[23]

There is also a danger that mammography will cause cancer due to the radiation used.[24] I have brought this to the attention of some doctors and nurses, and in all cases, the response has been that the radiation dose of a mammogram is harmless. However, radiation is radiation, and the accumulation over the years could most definitely cause damage.

---

22   "Breast Cancer Early Detection and Diagnosis," American Cancer Society, accessed August 10, 2020, https://www.cancer.org/cancer/breast-cancer/screening-tests-and-early-detection.html.

23   *Heal Breast Cancer Naturally*, p. 229.

24   Dr. Veronique Desaulniers, *Heal Breast Cancer Naturally* (Granger, Indiana: TCK Publishing, 2014) p. 229.

Unfortunately, some screenings are not covered by health insurance, but paying out of pocket might be worth it in the long run.

This reminds me of a quote by A. J. Reb Materi, a Catholic clergyman. "So many people spend their health gaining wealth and then have to spend their wealth to regain their health."

When it comes to paying for a screening test or paying a buck more for organic food, I know that investing in my well-being is the best investment I can do in life—for my life.

In summary, make every effort to prevent cancer or any other chronic degenerative condition. To do that, eat nutritious food, including brussels sprouts, cantaloupe, sweet potato, leafy greens such as spinach and kale, broccoli, blueberries, strawberries, pomegranates, bell peppers and mushrooms. Drink enough clean water; breathe deeply; and rest, relax, and exercise.

If you are diagnosed with cancer, do not rush into treatment. Remember that most cancers are slow growing. Do a favor to your body and get the facts about your condition. If most cancers need about five years to develop, there is no need for you to get into treatment right away.

Identify the best cancer screenings or testing for your type of cancer. There are multiple options, so decide which one fits your condition best. Listen to your body and to God or whomever you believe in, and do not agree to standard cancer treatment without making an informed decision about all options available. Remember that you have the power. It's your body, and you will face the consequences of your choices, whether they are negative or positive.

CHAPTER 4

THE STANDARD TREATMENT: SURGERY, CHEMOTHERAPY, AND RADIATION

The day I was diagnosed with cancer, my doctor referred me to the surgeon and the oncologist, assuming there were no other treatment options. Once you get cancer, the one-size-fits-all approach is prescribed. Both radiation and surgery had terrible effects on my body.

The burning sensation of radiation was awful. The radiated area turned dark due to the burn, and it was itchy for over a month after treatment ended. Radiation therapy made me extremely tired. It may even result in sterility, which was not a problem for me but could be for younger adults.

More problematic for me was that the radiation damage to my colon necessitated and ileostomy and then a second surgery to reverse that procedure four months later.

Surgery had devastating side effects on me, starting with collateral damage to one of my kidneys. surgery. I struggled with most of those side effects for a couple of years before I could get on my feet again, and the reality is that some of them will affect me for the rest of my life.

I am grateful, though, since it could have been worse if I had completed chemotherapy. I am grateful to God that I was able to stand up for my health and reject chemotherapy.

When the doctor wrote the prescription and asked me to go to the front desk to schedule chemotherapy treatment, I had already acquired enough knowledge to understand what chemotherapy would do to my body. Most likely, my immune system would crash; I would become anemic, lethargic, nauseated, and prone to other infections. and I would lose my hair and lose weight. I was already a skinny person and had lost about thirty pounds during surgery and radiation treatment. I could only imagine how I would look and feel if I were to lose more weight. It had been a real struggle to get over surgery and radiation, and there was no way I would go through chemotherapy.

Have you ever heard the expression, "Garbage in, garbage out," coined by George Fuechsel, an early computer programmer? By poisoning my body with chemotherapy, the outcome promised to be awful.

I dedicated a countless number of hours researching alternative options to chemo, and fortunately, I found several. I learned, though, that alternative medicine is not a one-size-fits-all approach either, and I utilized several approaches specifically for my individual circumstances. Among them was consulting with the Hoxsey Bio Medical Center in Tijuana, Mexico. I also followed the protocol of Johanna Budwig, PhD (1908–2003), a well-known German biochemist who devised the cottage cheese and flaxseed-oil diet, which I will explain in a later chapter. I took vitamin D3, magnesium, iodine, probiotics, and enzymes. I utilized essential oils, drank Essiac tea, improved by diet, began an exercise regimen, reprogramed my emotional state, got a hyperbaric oxygenation treatment, utilized energy healing, adopted a comprehensive detoxification strategy, and much more.

If you have already gone through the standard cancer treatment and think it could be too late for you regain your health, do not worry; there is always hope. You, too, can find alternative, holistic, natural approaches to detoxify, repair your body, and boost your immune system. Your immune system is the first line of defense against any illness, and cancer is no exception.

At the biomedical clinic in Tijuana, I had the opportunity to talk with patients who had been told the medical field could do nothing for them. I met patients from all over the United States and from other countries who shared their success stories about the effectiveness of alternative cancer treatments. They were young people and older people. They had a variety of types of cancer. Many were already in remission; others were still receiving treatment; some were new patients. Those patients were individuals who, for the most part, did not accept a doctor's statement that "nothing else can be done" and sought alternative opportunities to heal their bodies.

MY EXPERIENCE WITH RADIATION

The oncologist ordered twenty-five rounds of radiation over a period of approximately five weeks. I had learned that the side effects were mostly burning, extreme fatigue, and itching when peeing, and I was hesitant about it, but my ignorance and fear led me to follow through with the doctor's orders.

My first appointment, to get me ready for the treatment, fell on my birthday. It was a lousy way to celebrate a birthday. The oncologist said the radiation therapy would shrink the tumor and would make surgery more successful. Apparently, the twenty-five sessions of radiation helped to reduce the tumor to about half its size.

I had hoped that the treatment would shrink the tumor enough that I would not need surgery, but that didn't happen. Going through radiation therapy was not a big deal at first, because the treatment itself is not painful. I got through the first week easily. However, during the second and third weeks, I began to feel tremendous fatigue and a burning sensation in the radiated area. There was also intense itching in the radiated area. I was basically in bed for most of the day due to excessive fatigue and tiredness; my skin in the radiated area and its surroundings turned a dark color. Fortunately, most of the superficial symptoms disappeared within a few weeks after treatment ended.

Once radiation treatment was completed, I went to see the surgeon, who said that I still needed surgery as anticipated, but I had to wait approximately two months to allow my radiation-damaged colon to heal a bit before I could undergo surgery. The surgery removed the cancerous growths, but it also caused an enormous amount of stress to my body, which I have described.

What is radiation? According to the National Cancer Institute, radiation therapy (also called radiotherapy) is a cancer treatment that uses high doses of radiation to kill cancer cells and shrink tumors. External radiation comes from a device that aims radiation at your cancer. The device is large and may be noisy. It does not touch you, but can move around you, sending radiation to a part of your body from many directions.

External radiation is used for local treatment, which means it treats a specific part of your body. For example, if you have cancer in your lungs, you will have radiation only to your chest, not to your whole body. Radiation therapy may be given before, during, or after these other treatments to improve the chances that treatment will work.[25]

The timing of radiation therapy depends on the type of cancer being treated and whether the goal of radiation therapy is to treat cancer or ease symptoms. Radiation not only kills or slows the growth of cancer cells, but it can also affect nearby healthy cells. Damage to healthy cells can

---

25   "Radiation Therapy to Treat Cancer," accessed July 22, 2020, https://www.cancer.gov/about-cancer/treatment/types/radiation-therapy.

cause side effects.[26]

Many people who get radiation therapy suffer from fatigue. It can happen straight away or come on slowly. People feel fatigued to different degrees. This was only one of the symptoms; there was also emotional distress to deal with.

According to WebMD, "Late side effects from radiation therapy take months and sometimes years to show up and usually don't go away. But not everyone will have them.

"These problems happen when radiation damages your body. For example, scar tissue can affect the way your lungs or your heart works. Bladder, bowel, fertility, and sexual problems can start after radiation to your belly or pelvis."[27]

MY THOUGHTS ON CHEMOTHERAPY

Chemotherapy contains powerful chemicals that are actually bad for humans. The toxins that are used to kill cancer cells also kill healthy body cells and cause damage to organs. This makes recuperation from a chemotherapy treatment extremely difficult. In addition, the same substance that kills cancer cells contains cancer-causing chemicals. Chemotherapy can actually induce new cancers.

It is true that chemotherapy kills cancer cells, but the problem is that it kills good cells as well. It leaves your body defenseless and prone to consequences like liver failure, kidney failure, pneumonia, and infections. Why would you do that to your body? One of the big problems with chemotherapy is that it does not kill tumor stem cells. It only kills the daughter cells, so consequently, cancer often comes back, and it often comes back more aggressively.[28]

---

26   "Radiation Therapy to Treat Cancer."
27   "What to Expect from Radiation Therapy," accessed July 22, 2020, https://www.web-md.com/cancer/what-to-expect-from-radiation-therapy#2.
28   *The Truth About Cancer*, p. 75.

When my oncologist prescribed the chemo the second time, I had already acquired sufficient knowledge to decide that I was not going to go through it. There was no way that I was going to put my body through such stress and poison it more. Radiation had already done enough damage. There are several reasons for not doing chemotherapy as a treatment for cancer, the main one being that it does not cure cancer. It kills cancer cells, but it does not discriminate between healthy cells and malignant cells. It kills cells indiscriminately.

CHAPTER 5

Get Control of Your Health or Face the Consequences

The patient should be made to understand that they must take charge of their own life. Don't take your body to the doctor as if he were a repair shop.

—Quentin Regestein, MD

During the cancer treatment procedure, a urinary blockage occurred, and eventually, it killed one of my kidneys. According to my nephrologist, it most likely occurred during colon surgery. Nobody noticed this until almost a year after surgery, although my lab work had shown elevated creatinine levels ever since the surgery. However, none of my doctors—my GI doctor, my primary care physician, my oncologist, or my urologist—detected this early on, so my kidney could not be saved. It wasn't until I became concerned about having consistently elevated creatinine levels that I asked my primary care doctor to refer me to a kidney specialist. For about a year, every time this doctor reviewed my most updated lab work, he told me to drink more water because most likely, dehydration was the main reason for the elevated creatinine level.

The kidney specialist ordered a CT scan. This imaging technique uses X-rays to picture the kidneys. It may also be used to look for structural abnormalities and the presence of obstructions. It requires the use of intravenous contrast dye. The results were really demoralizing. One of my kidneys was working fine, but the other was only functioning at 3 percent. It was already too late to do anything about this, but what the urologist said intrigued me. "Many people can live with just one kidney," he said. "Do not worry about it."

Honestly, learning about my renal condition was devastating, especially because I had already experienced a family tragedy related to kidney failure. My stepdad had been on dialysis for about ten years due to kidney dysfunction, and I had seen firsthand how difficult the dialysis procedure was. It was very scary just thinking about the possibility of going through it.

I know there is a reason for having two kidneys, and I know the urologist's statement is true: there are a lot of individuals who live a normal life with one kidney. But I never should have had to face the challenge of having a damaged kidney because of medical negligence. Although drinking water is very important for the human body to function optimally, lack of water was not the reason for my kidney malfunction. It was negligence. Of course, no one would take responsibility for that, nor did I want to take it any further. Unfortunately, the kidney was irreparably damaged.

I am sharing this so you will be aware that you need to be on top of your medical conditions, because some doctors just look at patients superficially and do not delve into the situation thoroughly enough to see underlying issues. Apparently, for many doctors, patients are just numbers. They are working based on volume, not quality. Insurance companies are also to be blamed because several of them contract with doctors in a network and negotiate a rate per patient, which is usually lower than a doctor would charge for a consultation. Consequently, some doctors have to see many more patients to make up for that discounted price. In the long run, insurance companies often end up paying more, because the patient keeps going back to the doctor—in many cases, due to the poor quality of service the physician is providing.

That was my experience with some of the doctors I consulted during my journey to healing from cancer. I often had to wait an hour or two to be seen by the doctor, who would then spend about five minutes with me.

If even one of my doctors—the general doctor, the colon surgeon, the oncologist, or the urologist—had connected the fact that I'd just had colon surgery and radiation therapy to the red flag of elevated creatinine levels, my kidney might have been saved.

The doctors could have questioned why my kidney lab results were out of range or even why my blood pressure had been higher than usual since the surgery. My nephrologist said those variables were signals that the kidney was going through some problems. If doctors would give patients the time needed to really evaluate the medical conditions and analyze the whys and possible solutions, hundreds of cases of medical malpractice suits could be avoided. Fortunately, I discovered my kidney problem before it was too late to take better care of my other kidney. Do you know that medical care could be the third-leading cause of death in the United States?[29]

So, it is imperative for you to be careful and take control of your wellness. *You* are the person most interested in getting you healed. It is your responsibility to get a second or even third opinion. If you don't feel that you are getting the best medical treatment, then please go to another place.

---

29   Michael Greger MD, *How Not to Die* (London: Pan MacMillan, 2015) p. 251.

It is important to note that for cancer and other chronic conditions, a family member, friend, or other support person should accompany you on office visits. When you are the patient, stress can impair your capacity to think clearly and make sound decisions. Much of what I learned in my journey through healing cancer, I learned the hard way. I learned through trial and error.

I want to make the point that when I refer to "careless doctors," this statement is a generalization. I know there are many excellent doctors, and I deeply respect and honor for their commitment and passion. Still, you must be responsible for your own well-being and find those excellent doctors.

Many of us place too much trust in the medical profession. This is understandable, because after all, doctors spend years and years in school. Who are we to challenge their diagnoses and prescribed treatments? Fortunately, there are many well-trusted internet sites, books, and studies to read to become educated about your condition. I understand that the standard protocols for some illnesses are universal, but I am a firm believer that your unique conditions—such as lifestyle, age, environmental factors, and genes—make each case special. Do not accept the first diagnosis as a definitive one. Do not go blindly into a treatment.

In his book *The 9 Steps to Keep the Doctor Away*, Dr. Rashid A. Buttar writes: "

There are key moments in life when you are faced with a huge decision—one that will dramatically impact your future and the lives of those around you. In rare instances, your decision could impact the entire world. Some refer to such moments as 'crossroads,' and the intensity and challenge we feel at these moments can be a wake-up call for radical change. This is especially true in the sense that these metaphorical crossroads may present us with more than two distinct choices: We can accept the conventional paths, which are quite often the 'easy' solution. Or we can challenge the norm and take the road less traveled.[30]

Taking the road less traveled is painful for many of us. Most of us would hesitate to take this road. Most of us do what everybody does, regardless of the outcome.

For example, most people with diabetes believe that insulin is their savior. They *could* prevent or control their disease with recommended eating choices, exercise, rest, and stress reduction, but many keep doing the same things that predisposed them to diabetes in the first place. And if that's the only change they make to fix diabetes, they often end up moving to insulin injections and then needing dialysis treatment, as kidney disfunction is one of the domino effects of diabetes.

The same goes for other illnesses, such as cancer. Most cancer patients are rushed into the standard treatment of radiation, surgery, and chemotherapy without considering other possible options. It is very understandable that taking the less-traveled road could be challenging. You could face a lot of resistance from well-intentioned family members and friends, but if the facts are telling you that the conventional paths won't deliver positive results, then why not choose the less-traveled road, particularly if it is very promising? A cancer cure does not seem likely to be available any time soon. Just consider the following:

On December 23, 1971, President Richard Nixon signed the National Cancer Act of 1971 into law, launching the national war on cancer. Almost fifty years later, President Obama signed the High Mortality Cancer Bill into law as part of the National Defense Authorization Act of 2013. The bill requires the National Cancer Institute to "develop scientific frameworks for addressing cancers with survival rates of less than 50%, with first priority attention to lung and pancreatic cancers."[31]

---

30   Rashid A. Buttar, *The 9 Steps to Keep the Doctor Away* (Lake Tahoe, Nevada: GMEC Publishing, 2010), p. 4.

31   H.R. 4310, National Defence Authorization Act, January 2, 2012, https://www.govinfo. gov/content/pkg/BILLS-112hr4310enr/pdf/BILLS-112hr4310enr.pdf.

Since 1971, billions of dollars have been spent on trying to find the cure for cancer. But the rate of cancer remission is ridiculously low for most types of cancer, with the survival rate averaging five years. There is still no cure for cancer.

It is unbelievable that we have progressed in so many areas of science and technology and the world is changing at a speed never recorded before, but there is no cure for cancer! What to do? When it comes to your health, you have to take control into your own hands. Research your options. Look into alternative ways to cure your illness. Consider comprehensive approaches, because most likely you do not have cancer for just one reason. Do not sit and wait; get up and move, get hydrated, manage your stress levels, get seven to eight hours of sleep every night, eat a plant-based diet. These are basic principles. Do not think there is a magic pill to cure cancer or any other degenerative disease.

For any illness to develop, there is a series or a group of contributing factors. This is particularly true for cancer. When I developed colon cancer, it was not because I needed to eat more fiber, or I needed to drink more water. It wasn't because of my genes or because I was stressed or had a sedentary life or had too many toxins in my body. It wasn't because of any single factor. It was due to a combination of factors, and treating it required a combination of approaches.

I had to utilize several approaches to help my body regain wellness. After surgery and radiation, my health deteriorated even more. I had to fight for myself and find ways to support my body in the recovery process. In subsequent chapters, I will detail the approaches I utilized to get my body into balance and regain my health.

CHAPTER 6

A LEARNING EXPERIENCE

The best and most efficient pharmacy is within your own system.
—ROBERT C. PEALE

When I consulted the oncologist about my diagnosis and recommendations for treatment, he prescribed chemotherapy in tablet form to be taken concurrently with radiation. When he said that, my heart sank. I was more afraid of the chemotherapy than of cancer itself.

To me, chemotherapy was the reason for many cancer patients' dull appearance. I had already seen cancer patients undergoing chemotherapy, and it was heartbreaking to see how they looked. I could only imagine they felt even worse than their weak, pale, dull appearance showed.

I literally connected being under treatment with being at the end of my life. I remember grabbing the prescription and heading home. I cried and went into complete denial about needing that awful treatment.

After some thought, I decided not to take the pills. I continued with the radiation treatment by itself. A couple of weeks into the radiotherapy, I saw the oncologist for a follow-up appointment, and he asked me why I hadn't filled the chemotherapy prescription.

I responded, "Because I did not want to take them. I am afraid of the side effects."

He seemed upset and tried to persuade me to take them, saying that radiation would be more effective if administered concurrently with chemo. Out of confusion, I told him that I would go back to the pharmacy, fill the prescription, and follow his instructions. I was still hesitant to take the pills, but a question lingered in my mind: What if he was right?

But my instinct, hunch, gut feeling, or whatever you want to call it was *not* to take them. I continued with the radiation treatment without chemo.

After radiation therapy was concluded, I went to see the oncologist again. The next step was surgery. Two months later, I underwent a five-hour colon surgery, and at the same time, the surgeon put an ileostomy in my stomach. I was hospitalized for a week. After few weeks of recovery, I consulted with the oncologist again at a previously scheduled appointment. I remember that he flipped some pages of my medical record and asked me a couple of questions about the ileostomy. Then he said that I needed to talk to my surgeon, because I would need to have the ileostomy removed sooner than scheduled, so I could start chemotherapy treatment.

I asked him why he was prescribing chemotherapy. I was particularly interested because he did not do any follow-up blood work or other testing regarding my specific type of cancer or the type of chemotherapy "suited" for my condition.

I was confused by this directive, because my Cancer (CA) marker test, which according to my oncologist, should be below 2.5 for a colon cancer patient, was within the normal range.

The reason he gave me was: "This is part of the treatment regimen in case there are still some malignant cells in the bloodstream." Thank God I refused chemotherapy again, and those "left-over malignant cells" were taken care of with natural approaches.

He did not offer any explanation about what kind of chemotherapy would be administered, nor did he take the time to explain the facts or data-driven reasons for the treatment. I expected a sounder reason than "because it's part of the treatment regimen."

According to the Centers for Disease Control and Prevention, in 2015, the latest year for which incident data are available, 1,633,390 new cases of cancer were reported, and 595,919 people died of cancer in the United States. For every 100,000 people, 438 new cases were reported and 159 died of cancer. This data is pretty scary.[32]

The number of people being diagnosed with cancer every year is extremely high. However, the five-year relative survival rate for cancer in the United States is 65 percent, which seems fairly good. It must be mentioned here that this percentage does not reveal anything about the quality of life of cancer survivors who went through conventional treatment or of those who survived thanks to alternative treatments.

When the oncologist prescribed chemotherapy for me, I felt he was using the one-size-fits-all approach to treat cancer. By then, I had already learned that some doctors—even those who prescribe the standard treatment—go above and beyond the one-size-fits-all treatment and really take the time to analyze which kind of chemo would work for a specific type and stage of cancer.

All I remember him telling me is that I was going to receive chemotherapy through a port that would be inserted in my chest, and I would have the port for twelve weeks, which would be the length of the treatment. Then he directed me to the receptionist to schedule my appointment

---

32   "United States Cancer Statistics: Highlights from 2015 Incidence," Centers for Disease Control and Prevention, https://www.cdc.gov/cancer/uscs/about/data-briefs/no3-USCS-highlights-2015-incidence.htm.

to have the port inserted in my chest. Those were the last words I heard from him.

Instead of going to the receptionist to schedule the follow-up appointment, I left his office and never went back. I hesitated to undergo chemotherapy for many reasons. The first was that I had friends and relatives who had already gone through chemotherapy, and most of them were dead.

I had seen and read enough about this type of one-size-fits-all cancer treatment approach to understand that it would hurt me more than help me. Yes, it would kill cancer cells, but it would also kill good cells. Killing healthy cells leaves your body vulnerable to other problems, including organ damage, infections, and a weak immune system.

I knew I refusing chemotherapy was the right decision for me. However I have to admit, I was fearful, too. My mind was in turmoil because most of the publicly accepted information that I had from Western medicine was that chemotherapy was the only accepted method of treating cancer. Therefore, the decision to not go through chemo was challenging.

Based on my awareness of other available options and the knowledge I had acquired through reading books and other research—including the fact that the success rate for standard treatment was low for most types of cancer—the cons outweighed the benefits, and I decided to say no to chemo once and for all.

I was convinced that chemotherapy wouldn't heal my body but would only damage it more. I was also convinced that by following a healthy lifestyle, including detoxifying my body, eating nutritious food, exercising, and managing my stress levels, I would be in a better position than with chemotherapy. Fortunately, my husband agreed and supported my decision, which made the journey easier.

Since I had left the doctor thinking that I would do chemo, I received several phone calls from his office trying to schedule my next appointment. I asked them to stop calling me because I was not going to accept the treatment.

Still, I needed to continue monitoring the cancer, so I decided to see a new oncologist for my regular checkups to monitor my overall wellness. That experience was different because I was not a cancer patient anymore. I was a patient in "remission." Thanks to God and to brave, caring people in the "alterative field," I was learning methods for taking care of my health. As of this writing, I have been cancer free for six years now, without chemotherapy.

I am healthier than ever and happy and grateful to God for giving me the opportunity to continue living and for giving me a second chance.

Cancer was a turning point in my life. It gave me another perspective on life and taught me the importance of giving my best self to what matters most.

Although the oncologist did not mention these to me, I've compiled a list of typical chemotherapy side effects from different sources. They include but are not limited to: fatigue, decreased white blood cell count, increased risk of infection that can land you in the hospital and may be life-threatening, abdominal cramping, constipation, a compromised immune system, weight loss, loss of appetite, weakness, damaged DNA, and neuropathy, such as numbness or tingling in your hands or feet or a loss of sensation.[33]

It all depends on the type of chemotherapy and your general wellness condition. The oncologist said that I would get some peeling on my fingers and I would lose hair, although it grows back once treatment is over. As you can see, the list goes on and on. I am so glad that I decided not to undergo chemotherapy.

---

33   "Get ready for possible side effects of chemotherapy." Updated November 1, 2018, https://www.mayoclinic.org/tests-procedures/chemotherapy/about/pac-20385033

CHAPTER 7

Let's Talk about Excess in Your Body

Detoxification is a natural process that must occur in your body order for any health intervention to work properly. Allowing toxins to accumulate in your body is similar to running a central air-conditioning system with a dirty filter; it forces the unit to work harder and increases the risk that the system will break down. Our bodies have several natural filter systems, but if they are forced to work overly hard to get rid of toxins, they won't be able to aid the healing process.

Detoxification is more important than ever. As Ilse Marie Issels writes on the website Issels Immuno-Oncology:

No other generation before ours has been exposed to as many human-made chemicals and toxic substances as we are. The air we breathe is polluted; the water we drink is not clean; the food we eat is processed; the food for our souls is provided by a sensationalizing media; our lifestyle is sedentary; our cells lack oxygen, vitamins, minerals, and enzymes; our organs of detoxification and excretion are overwhelmed; and our bodies are overloaded with waste products and toxic metabolites, which render them vulnerable to all sorts of bacteria and viruses. How do we survive?[34]

Specifically, there are six organs and systems responsible for processing the constant barrage of toxins in our bodies. They are the main channels of detoxification, and each plays an important role. They act as filters, and keeping the filters clean is essential to proper organ function.[35] They are:

1. Gut
2. Liver
3. Lungs
4. Kidneys
5. Skin
6. Lymphatic system

In our modern world, these organs/systems are overwhelmed by the number of toxins in our bodies—it's been estimated that we carry over 700 contaminants in our body at any one time regardless of whether we live in a big city or a rural area. According to the Organic Grace website, "Because many chemicals have the ability to attach to dust particles and/or catch air and water currents and travel far from where they are produced or used, the globe is bathed in a chemical soup. Our bodies have no alternative but to absorb these chemicals and sometimes store them for long periods of time."[36] Simply put, your hardworking detox organs need a helping hand!

Let's look into the role of each organ and system and the simple things you can do to make sure they are able to process toxins at an optimal level.

---

34   Ilse Marie Issels, "Information on Detoxification," 2001, accessed July 22, 2020, https://issels.com/publication-library/information-on-detoxification/.

35   "Information on Detoxification."

36   "The Body Burden," Organic Grace website, accessed July 22, 2020, https://organic-grace.com/body-burden.

THE GUT

The gut, consisting of the esophagus, stomach, intestines, and colon, is the first defender against toxins that you ingest. Several research studies support the fact that the condition of your GI tract—specifically, the health of your colon—is highly correlated with that of your immune system. Colorectal cancer is the "third most common cancer diagnosed in both men and women in the United States," according to the American Cancer Society. The ACS makes the following projections for 2020:

- 104,610 new cases of colon cancer
- 43,340 new cases of rectal cancer[37]

In *Beating Cancer with Nutrition*, Dr. Quillin explains that 40 percent of your immune system surrounds the gastrointestinal tract, and he stresses the importance of a strong immune system as a critical aspect of health.[38]

When your gut is well-balanced, it draws essential nutrients from what you eat and drink and leaves toxins in the gastrointestinal tract to be eliminated. But if you don't have healthy bacteria in your gut or there is a blockage, then toxins linger in your body and perhaps become absorbed.

To keep your gut functioning optimally, try these tips from nutrition expert Dr. Deanna Minich:

Eat more fiber: Root vegetables, gluten-free grains, and other high-fiber foods mechanically clear toxins from the body by "scraping" toxins out of the gut and through the colon for elimination.

Try probiotics: Certain types of probiotics called lactobacilli have been shown to eliminate carcinogens from the body and absorb heavy metals. Lactobacilli are found in fermented dairy foods like yogurt and kefir, as well as in fermented dairy-free foods like miso and tempeh. You can also take probiotics with lactobacillus as a supplement in pill form.

---

37   "Key Statistics for Colorectal Cancer," updated January 23, 2020, https://www.cancer.org/cancer/colon-rectal-cancer/about/key-statistics.html.

38   *Beating Cancer with Nutrition*, p. 107.

Drink water: To detoxify your colon, drink plenty of water. You will see this suggestion in most articles related to health, nutrition, detoxification, and hydration because water is essential to the overall functioning of the body.

Move your bowels regularly: The liver sends toxic metabolic waste into the colon to be eliminated when you move your bowels, so it is important to be regular. Typically, you should poop the same number of times you eat—two or three times a day. The more you defecate, the more you eliminate toxins.

Maintaining your colon functioning at optimal levels requires a lifestyle that supports it. Eating food with high fiber content, drinking enough water, and eating fruits and vegetables are not something you do once and then you're done. That would be just like trying to lose weight by eating healthy only once a week. It simply doesn't work that way. As hard as it may sound, you need to stay the course.[39]

THE LIVER

The liver performs many vital digestive and hormonal tasks—it is responsible for the proper functioning of the body in general. Among its tasks is detoxification. The liver, along with the kidneys, detoxifies your blood by filtering toxins from the blood and eliminating toxins that arise during digestion.

This metabolic waste could be related to something you ate or produced by normal cell activity. It all needs to go. It's like the filter on your air-conditioning unit: you have to change the filter periodically, so it doesn't become clogged. If it's clogged, your air conditioner has to work harder until eventually, it breaks. Similarly, if you don't help maintain your liver and kidneys by choosing beneficial foods, eventually those filters will be overloaded and their ability to work properly will diminish. The website Medical News Today provides a list of foods that help keep

---

39   Dr. Deanna Minich, "Modern-Day Ways to Support Your 5 Detox Organs," Dr. Deanna Minich website, October 14, 2016, https://www.deannaminich.com/5-detox-organs/.

your liver heathy. People should eat these foods as part of a whole and balanced diet. They include:

- oatmeal
- green tea
- garlic
- berries
- nuts
- avocados
- bananas
- barley
- beets and beet juice
- broccoli
- brown rice
- carrots
- figs
- greens such as kale and collards
- lemons
- papayas
- watermelon[40]

In *Beating Cancer with Nutrition*, Dr. Patrick Quillin recommends milk thistle, also known as silybum marianum, to help detoxify the liver, writing, "Its seeds, fruit and leaves are widely prescribed medication in Europe for most diseases affecting the liver."[41]

You will most likely see that some foods that are beneficial for your liver are also beneficial for your colon and your health in general. That's because if you eat healthy "real" food, you will see synergistic results.

---

40   Jon Johnson, "What foods protect the liver?" Medical News Today, January 23, 2020, https://www.medicalnewstoday.com/articles/323915.

41   *Beating Cancer with Nutrition*, p. 229.

THE LUNGS

We can live a few weeks without food, a few days without water, but only a few minutes without air. Lung cancer in the number-one killer of all cancers, according Dr. Michael Greger, author of *How Not to Die*. Do not take for granted the fact that you can breathe!

Ease the load on your lungs with these tips:

Invest in an air filter: At the beginning of the chapter, I talked about how toxic our environment is. It basically does not matter where in the world we live; we inhale many toxins with every breath—dust, exhaust fumes, pesticides, insecticides, factory emissions, and more. It is almost impossible to control what is happening in the outdoor environment, but what we can do is invest in an air filter for our homes. An air filter will do part of the filtering work your lungs would do, reducing the burden on them.

Exercise in clean air: If you exercise outdoors, choose a place with cleaner air, such as a forest or park with lots of trees rather than a city neighborhood. Reducing the amount of pollutants that enter your lungs will give them a break.

Try deep-breathing exercises: The lungs have a simple and effective way of getting rid of toxins: breathing out! We can support this process by taking time every day to engage in deep breathing. Deep breathing also helps to release stress and shift you into a state of calmness. Dr. Becky Bailey's website, Conscious Discipline, contains one of my favorite deep-breathing models. It is family oriented and involving other family members is a powerful practice. According to Bailey, "Three deep breaths shut off the 'fight or flight' system of the brain. This active calming technique is an essential component of emotional health. Teach children to STAR: Smile, Take a deep breath, And Relax."[42]

---

42   Conscious Discipline website, accessed July 23, 2020, https://consciousdiscipline.com/free-resources/shubert/shuberts-classroom/s-t-a-r/.

I recommend doing deep-breathing exercises on the "four-by-four" schedule—that is, four cycles, four times a day. Dr. Edward Group describes the following method on the Global Healing website:

> Find a relaxing and quiet place to sit down. Close your eyes and begin by breathing in deeply through your nose, from your belly up. Count to five, inhaling the entire time. Even when you think you can't inhale anymore, try to squeeze a little more air in. Allow your lungs and stomach to fully inflate.
>
> Hold your breath for several seconds and then exhale over the course of another five count. When you think you can't exhale any more, keep blowing from the deepest depths of your lungs and stomach. You should feel your chest and abdomen flatten inward.[43]

Performing this exercise daily will not only relieve stress, but it cleanses the lungs and allows for more oxygenation of the cells all over the body, which improves health, helps all the body's systems perform better, and even can provide you with more energy. Deep breathing also actually helps to stretch out the torso.

Oxygen is the miracle of life. How important is oxygen? The human body requires oxygen to make the energy that powers the brain and muscles. It turns genes on and off. It encourages waste removal. Oxygen stimulates blood vessel growth to heal wounds. If your cells become deprived of oxygen, they shut down and begin to die. Bottom line: your body won't function without oxygen.

---

43   Dr. Edward Group, "Deep Breathing for Lung Cleansing," Global Healing, updated August 8, 2014, https://globalhealing.com/natural-health/deep-breathing-for-lung-cleansing/#:~:text=This%20allows%20for%20more%20oxygenation%20of%20the%20cells,very%20large%20torsos%20to%20see%20this%20in%20action.

THE KIDNEYS

The kidneys are among the main organs of detoxification, and they are essential for the body's functioning. When I found out about the damage one of my kidneys had suffered during the cancer treatment, it was devastating for me, because I know how important these organs are. Kidneys work nonstop cleaning toxins from your blood.

According to Dr. Michael Greger, the kidneys "process about 150 quarts of blood every 24 hours just to make the 1-2 quarts of urine you pee out each day."[44] When they are not functioning properly, he writes in *How Not to Die*, a person may experience symptoms such as weakness and abnormal heart rhythm. No wonder I was feeling so tired! No wonder my blood pressure was consistently higher than normal (registering over 140 when a normal reading for me was 110).

Although the heart is not an organ that detoxifies the body, I mention the correlation between heart health and kidney health because it could be a lifesaver for you. High blood pressure is a silent killer. Elevated blood pressure can damage the kidneys, which in turn threatens the health of other organs. "Our kidneys are so critical to proper heart function that patients under age of forty-five with kidney failure can be a hundred times more likely to die of heart disease than those with working kidneys," according to Greger.[45]

The kidneys have several functions besides cleaning your blood. The kidneys also balance fluids in your body, which is important for circulation and for microbial balance. If your kidneys aren't functioning optimally, toxins can remain in circulation throughout the body, causing harm.

Do your kidneys a favor by staying well hydrated and eating whole, healthy foods. For kidney cleansing, the Advanced Urology Institute recommends the regular intake of apple cider vinegar, kidney beans,

---

44   *How Not to Die*, p. 165.
45   *How Not to Die*, p. 165.

lemon juice, watermelon, pomegranate, basil, dates, and fresh dandelion or dried dandelion brewed as tea.[46]

THE SKIN

Our skin is not just a cover for our bodies. The skin is our largest detox organ. It is designed to eliminate toxins through perspiration, but it can also absorb toxins. That's why it is important to watch what you put on your skin. You can help yourself by selecting natural body products. When you are choosing lotions, creams, sunscreen, and deodorant, one rule of thumb is to read the product labels, and if you do not understand them or cannot even pronounce the names of ingredients, do not use them. I personally use organic coconut oil as body lotion and as a makeup remover.

Sweating—one of the many benefits of exercise—is the best thing you can do for your skin. But consult with your healthcare providers before starting any exhaustive exercise regimen, particularly if you suffer from a chronic condition.

Another of my favorite skin-health practices is dry brushing, which helps to unclog pores and makes your skin glow. I have a discipline of dry brushing at least three times a week, and one result is the feeling of higher energy.

Dry brushing stimulates the lymphatic system to release toxins. The lymphatic cells dump metabolic waste into the lymph system, and the lymph system carries it to your liver and kidneys to eliminate it. Dry brushing also improves circulation and reduces cellulite.[47]

You always brush dry skin using a natural-bristled brush. You start with your feet and work up, brushing with a circular motion and making sure that you cover all areas of your body, including torso and back. A

---

46   "8 Easy Ways to Cleanse Your Kidneys," Advanced Urology Institute, October, 11, 2017, https://www.advancedurologyinstitute.com/8-easy-ways-cleanse-kidneys/.

47   "Dry Brushing: Benefits, Risks, and More," Healthline, September 29, 2017, https://www.healthline.com/health/dry-brushing.

couple of swipes in each area is sufficient. Do not go over an area too many times because it could cause irritation to your skin. Never brush skin that is irritated. (See chapter 9 for more information on dry brushing.)

THE LYMPH SYSTEM

Last but not least, the lymph system has a huge role in detoxification and defense. "About two liters of lymph fluid circulate in our lymphatic vessels, which cover the body from the tips of the toes to the top of the head. These two liters are formed continually from the interstitial fluid that is the extracellular fluid surrounding each one of our body cells."[48]

Most of us have experienced enlarged and painful "swollen glands" when we get sick. Lymphatic glands or nodes are located throughout the body. Their purpose is to produce white blood cells (aka "lymphocytes") to battle infections and invaders, according to Issels.com.

"If the production of lymphocytes is insufficient, the body's defense against invaders and against cancer and other immune disorders will be impaired. If the work of the lymph nodes is insufficient, the filtering, the degradation, and the transport of the waste products will be impeded, and the bodily environment will become overwhelmed with toxic metabolites and toxins."[49] I had never thought about the lymphatic system until I began researching ways to heal my body from cancer. I discovered how important it is to detoxify the lymphatic system. Luckily, an exercise as simple as rebounding—jumping on a tiny trampoline--works fine. (More on rebounding in chapter 9.)

A BRIEF DISCUSSION OF HEAVY METALS

Heavy metals like mercury and aluminum are dangerous and cancer-causing. In his book *The 9 Steps to Keep the Doctor Away*, Dr. Rashid Buttar

---

48   "The Lymph System and Detoxification," accessed July 23, 2020, https://issels.com/treatment/detoxification/lymphsystem.aspx.

49   "The Lymph System and Detoxification."

talks about the importance of monitoring your diet and environment for heavy metals and avoiding them, if possible. Many vaccines like the flu shot contain heavy mercury as thimerosal. Other products we consume, such as tuna, are polluted with mercury. Aluminum, another toxic metal, can be found in cheese and canned meats as sodium aluminum phosphate. If you have silver fillings in your mouth, 50 percent of that material is mercury, and mercury is a cancer causer.[50] Find a holistic dentist to remove your silver filings.

One more thing. What about your cleaning supplies? I only use baking soda, vinegar, and soap to clean my entire house and essential oils for aromatizing.

Removing pollutants from our environments and detoxifying our bodies are important steps in working toward beating cancer and achieving wellness in general. Do these processes take effort? Sure. But as Stephen Covey, author of *The Seven Habits of Highly Effective People* states, "The successful person has the habit of doing the things failures don't like to do."

---

50   Dr. Rashid Buttar, *The 9 Steps to Keep the Doctor Away* (Lake Tahoe, Nevada: GMEC Publishing, 2010.

CHAPTER 8

Nutrition

Let food be thy medicine and medicine be thy food.
—Hippocrates

I am not a nutritionist. My advice is based on my own experience. But I promise you, learning to eat healthier food helped me regain wellness and energy. Friends and family commented on my speedy recovery and attributed it to my better eating habits.

Change is an interesting process. As you might know, we are often very resistant to it. After I was diagnosed with cancer, I found myself reading everything I could about nutrition and discovered several different approaches. It was difficult to decide which one to use, since most of them made a lot of sense.

It seems logical to give your body what it needs to fight illness, to become aware of your present health situation, and to analyze your past and current eating habits. There are questions to ponder when it comes to your wellness. For example, are you eating to nourish your body or are you eating to satiate your hunger? There is a great difference between these two concepts.

Many people tend to believe that because they are chubby, they are healthy. But that's not necessarily true. Although there are exceptions to the rule, most junk-food eaters are not healthy or eventually become ill. There is only so much the body can handle before it runs on empty and health problems arise.

Becoming aware of what are you putting into your mouth is the cornerstone of good health. Becoming educated about food nutrients is necessary because many foods lack necessary nutrients. Luckily, a ton of reliable information is available.

It is important to learn about balancing the diet. Complete meals include necessary nutrients and a balance between protein and carbohydrates.

Deciding to make better eating choices was a no-brainer for me because the facts were clear. For the first three years, I was hardcore about sticking to my healthy eating habits. But maintaining consistent habits has been extremely hard. It's still a challenge to see family members and friends eating more appealing food and having to decide between tasty or healthy. That is not to say that healthy food is not tasty, but a change to your diet is also a challenge to your palate.

I encourage you to work with a family member or friend and challenge and support each other to eat healthier.

Believe me, I understand that changing habits takes a lot of determination, persistence, and consistency. But it is rewarding to see the changes when new habits aimed at supporting your overall wellness become evident. You will notice the benefits in your skin, your hair, your weight, and your general wellness.

> The doctor of the future will no longer treat the human frame with drugs but will rather cure and prevent disease with nutrition.
>
> —Thomas Edison

EAT REAL FOOD

One hundred years ago, Thomas Alva Edison, an American inventor and businessman, was aware of the importance of proper nutrition. Yet orthodox medicine still utilizes medication as the main method of treating illness. It is up to us to take responsibility for our health through better nutrition. Do not wait until it is too late to understand that poor eating habits could be cutting your life short.

On the website GettingHealthier.com, Dr. Patrick Quillin reiterates the common-sense notion that we are what we eat. And for many of us, that is bad news. He writes:

Veterinarians know the irreplaceable link between nutrient intake and the health of the animals they care for. Actually, most pets and zoo creatures eat better than most Americans do. Your dog or cat probably gets a balanced formula of protein, carbohydrates, fat, fiber vitamins, and minerals…yet most of us eat for taste, cost, emotional needs, and convenience. The most commonly eaten food in America is heavily refined and nutritionally bankrupt white flour. Meanwhile, our livestock eats the more nutritious wheat germ and bran that we discard. When our crops are not doing well, we examine the soil for nutrients, fluid, and pH content. Our gardens prosper when we water, fertilize, and add a little broad-spectrum mineral supplement such as Miracle Gro to them. A sign posted near the junk food vending machines in a major city zoo warns: "Do not feed this food to animals or they might get sick and die." [51]

Think about it! Why is it that junk food isn't to be given to animals, but it is served in schools and hospitals? Why is it that our most vulnerable population, sick people, is allowed to eat what animals should not?

When I was in the hospital recuperating from surgery, I was graciously offered snacks in between meals. They were usually ice cream and fruit juice packed with sugar and artificial flavors and colors. I began to think about how lacking in nutrients those snacks were, particularly for a weak body like mine was back then. Nutrition is one of the lowest priorities in most orthodox health-care institutions, but it should be the basis of wellness.

There are currently more obese people than ever before. It's difficult to understand why institutions like schools and hospitals, which are regulated by the government, do not emphasize the importance of nutrition as a form of prevention. I will leave that question for you to ponder. But you can make a difference for yourself and your immediate family.

When I read Dr. Quillin's beautifully written book, *Beating Cancer with Nutrition*, it was a turning point for me. It was unbelievable to realize that I was neglecting one of the most important aspects of my health.

Changing my diet was challenging because my body was used to my lifelong eating habits. I had to learn to buy most of my food from the produce section and avoid the aisles of the grocery stores where all the flour-based and sugary stuff is displayed.

I also avoided buying canned food, because the canned food contains lots of sodium and preservatives in addition to BPA.

According to the Mayo Clinic, BPA stands for bisphenol A, and it is an industrial chemical that has been used to make certain plastics and resins since the 1960s.[52] You need to reduce your use of canned foods,

---

51   Patrick Quillin, "Can the Mediterranean Diet Reverse Disease?" Getting Healthier website, December 16, 2018, https://gettinghealthier.com/can-nutrition-reverse-disease/.
52   "What is BPA?" Mayo Clinic, https://www.mayoclinic.org/healthy- lifestyle/nutrition-and-healthy-eating/expert-answers/bpa/ faq-20058331.

since most cans are lined with BPA-containing resin. According to the Natural Resources Defense Council (NRDC) BPA is toxic. "It's used in the lining of food and soda cans to prevent the contents from corroding the metal. BPA also serves as a 'developer' in thermal paper receipts."[53]

It is amazing that this information is not shared with the public. Public-health agencies should create massive campaigns to inform the public, particularly parents so they can avoid giving to their children this poison. Understanding this was of tremendous help to me. I no longer buy any canned food, unless it explicitly states it is BPA free.

I modified my diet from a high-carb, sugar-filled diet to a leaner one. That meant that during the hardcore treatment period, I had to remove food items containing flour, including bread, pasta, and tortillas, from my table. In the beginning, I excluded a lot of items, such as starchy food, flour, sugar, and lactose, and incorporated into my diet a lot of vegetables and fruits, making sure that I was eating enough protein. This was particularly challenging for me because I have never been a heavy meat eater. But getting educated about food that contains protein other than meat was a task I had to accomplish. Besides meat, you can also find protein in the following foods, among others: eggs, almonds, oats, broccoli, tuna, quinoa, lentils, Ezekiel bread, and Brussels sprouts.

Before cancer, my vegetable intake was limited to just a few items. To change that lifetime habit, I would try one new vegetable at a time and try to prepare it in different ways—juiced, steamed, raw, etc. Although I was not a regular "junk food" eater, my diet was extremely high in carbs such as rice, potatoes, and flour. Basically, my body was still craving carbs as I tried to shift to "whole foods" like fruits and vegetables.

I learned to avoid the aisle/middle sections of supermarkets, where most of the heavily processed foods are displayed. I was applying the

---

53   "4 Ways to Avoid Toxic Chemicals in Food Packaging," Natural Resources Defense Council, August 12, 2015, https://www.nrdc.org/stories/4-ways-avoid-toxic-chemicals-food-packaging.

out-of-sight out-of-mind concept by not exposing myself to the temptation of high-carbohydrate foods.

Instead, I bought denser, nutrient-rich vegetables such as broccoli, cauliflower, and cabbage. I would be creative with the preparation of these to add variety to my meals. I chose fruits with lower glycemic index like pomegranates, blueberries, and raspberries, although in smaller qualities I would also consume other fruits like bananas, figs, dates, and dark grapes. One of my all times favorite dishes was oatmeal loaded with nuts and berries. To assist my gastrointestinal tract, I also drank kefir almost every day.

A meta-analysis study published in the *Journal of the American College and Nutrition* found that fruit and vegetable supplements also confer health benefits. "Overall, daily consumption of fruits and vegetable (FV) supplements significantly increased serum concentrations of the major antioxidant provitamins and vitamins found in plant foods (β-carotene, vitamins C and E) and folate."[54]

My sole intention was to give my body what it needed to heal itself. Once I learned to identify food nutrients from labels and/or from literature, it all began to make more sense to me, and having this information helped me to stay the course. The testimonies of people who had acquired optimal wellness through nutrition also helped and encouraged me.

People who eat seven or more portions of fresh fruits and vegetables each day may reduce their risk of dying from a wide variety of diseases by as much as 42 percent compared with people who consume less than one portion, according to a study by British researchers who tracked the eating habits of more than 65,000 people for twelve years.[55]

More remarkably, the researchers said they were able to quantify the health benefits per portion of fruits and vegetables consumed. One

---

54   Amin Esfahani, "Health effects of mixed fruit and vegetable concentrates: a systematic review of the clinical interventions," *Journal of the American College of Nutrition* vol. 20,5 (2011), p. 285294.

55   Ben Radding, "More Veggies Could Save your Life," Men's Journal, accessed July 23, 2020, https://www.mensjournal.com/food-drink/more-veggies-could-save-your-life/.

to three portions daily reduced the chance of death from any cause by 14 percent, three to five portions had a 29 percent impact, five to seven portions dropped the chances by 36 percent, and seven or more portions produced a 42 percent decline in the risk of death. The benefits appeared to tail off at that level.[56] Isn't that amazing? To think that we can increase the possibility of living a longer and healthier life by consuming more fresh fruits and vegetables.

JUICING

Juice was and continues to be my primary source of energy. I started juicing every day, and I still juice at least five days a week. Juicing is the process of extracting juice from fruit, vegetables, or tubers. The juice can be extracted using any one of a growing number of juicing machines on the market, including hand juicers, masticating juicers, twin juicers, hydraulic press juicers, and centrifugal juicers.

The resultant nutrient-rich liquid is usually consumed immediately after juicing to maximize the health benefits.

Although fresh juice contains the same nutrients as the original fruits and vegetables, the juicing process removes fibers and makes the juice more concentrated. It is easier to digest and easier to absorb into the bloodstream.

Consequently, juicing is a more effective way to absorb high concentrations of nutrients (vitamins, minerals, and enzymes) from fruits and vegetables into the body. This was a cornerstone of my recuperation.

Organic fruits and vegetables are highly recommended for juicing—unfortunately, most nonorganic fruits and vegetables are contaminated with herbicides and pesticides.

If possible, it would be best to grow your own fruits and vegetables or at least buy season fruits and vegetables from local growers. That's because

---

56   "More Veggies Could Save your Life."

most of the fruits and vegetables from grocery stores are harvested when they are still green so they can be transported without spoiling.

After radiation and surgery, my body was debilitated. The side effects of those procedures had sent me to the ground. From there, thanks to God and to all the learning I did, I managed to get back onto my two feet. I am very thankful to my family members, particularly my husband, for supporting me in this journey.

The following list of fruits and vegetables and their nutritional values comes from the Healthline website:

- Carrots are antibacterial, antifungal, anti-inflammatory, immune-boosting, and have anti-cancer properties, specifically against leukemia and colon cancer.

- Beets are high in antioxidants. Like carrots, they're also rich in carotenoids, lycopene, and vitamin A. Beets are also a good source of vitamin C, folate, manganese, and potassium. They can lower your blood pressure and even improve physical performance.

- Celery contains vitamins A, C, and K, as well as minerals like potassium, calcium, and magnesium, and some noteworthy anti-cancer flavonoids.

- Fresh bell peppers, red or green, are a rich source of vitamin C. This vitamin is particularly concentrated in red peppers. Just 100g of red pepper provides about 242mg of vitamin C, a potent water-soluble antioxidant. Inside the human body, it is required for collagen synthesis. Collagen is the main structural protein in the body required for maintaining the integrity of blood vessels, skin, organs, and bones. Regular consumption of foods rich in this vitamin prevents scurvy, boosts immunity, and scavenges harmful and inflammatory free radicals from the body.

- Cucumbers contain unique antioxidants in moderate amounts, such as vitamin C, vitamin A, zeaxanthin, and lutein. These compounds act as protective scavengers against oxygen-derived free radicals and reactive oxygen species (ROS) that play a role in aging and various disease processes. Cucumbers have a surprising amount of vitamin K and provide about 17 ug of this vitamin per 100 g. Vitamin K has been found to play a role in bone strength by promoting osteoblastic (bone mass building) activity. It also has an established role in the treatment of Alzheimer's disease by limiting neuronal damage in the human brain.

- The antioxidants present in tomatoes have been found to be protective against cancers, including colon, prostate, breast, endometrial, lung, and pancreatic tumors. Lycopene, a flavonoid antioxidant, is a unique phytochemical compound found in tomatoes. Red fruits tend to possess more of this antioxidant. Together with carotenoids, lycopene may help protect cells and other structures in the human body from harmful oxygen-free radicals. Studies show that lycopene protects the skin from ultra-violet (UV) rays and thus offers some defense against skin cancer. Zeaxanthin is another flavonoid compound present abundantly in this vegetable. It helps protect eyes from "age-related macular degeneration" (ARMD) in older adults by filtering harmful ultraviolet rays.

- Lemons are low in calories, having just 29 calories per 100g. They contain zero saturated fats or cholesterol. Nonetheless, they are an excellent source of dietary fiber (7.36 percent of RDA). Lemons are one of the very low glycemic fruits. Citric acid constitutes up to 8 percent of its juice. It is a natural preservative, aids in smooth digestion, and helps dissolve kidney stones. Lemons, like other citrus fruits, are an excellent source of the antioxidant vitamin C (ascorbic acid, which is helpful in preventing scurvy. Besides that, the consumption of foods rich in vitamin C helps the human body develop resistance against infectious agents and scavenge harmful, pro-inflammatory free radicals from the blood. Lemons also carry a healthy amount of minerals like iron, copper, potassium, and calcium. Potassium is an important component of cell and body fluids that helps control heart rate and blood pressure.

- Apples are rich in antioxidant phytonutrients, flavonoids, and polyphenolics. Some of the important flavonoids in apples are quercetin, epicatechin, and procyanidin B2. Additionally, they are also high in tartaric acid which is what gives them their tart flavor. Altogether, these compounds help protect the body from the harmful effects of free radicals. Apples contain good quantities of vitamin C and B-carotene.

- The avocado contains many health-promoting flavonoids and polyphenolic antioxidants such as cryptoxanthin, lutein, zeaxanthin, beta and alpha carotenes, albeit in small amounts. Together, these compounds work as protective scavengers against oxygen-derived free radicals and reactive oxygen species (ROS) that play a role in aging and various disease processes. Avocados are also high in many health-benefiting vitamins such as vitamins A, E, K. Avocados are also excellent sources of minerals like iron, copper, magnesium, and manganese. Magnesium is essential for bone strengthening and has a cardiac-protective role as well. Manganese is used by the human body as a co-factor for the antioxidant enzyme, superoxide dismutase. Iron and copper are required for the production of red blood cells.[57]

The list goes on and on. There are several reliable websites and books where you can find the nutritional values of almost any kind of fruit and vegetable that could be of help for your particular condition. There are so many options that it's easy to end up not doing anything. I started juicing with a cheap juicer that was complicated to use and to clean. Later, I

---

57   "Juicing: Good or Bad?" Healthline, October 4, 2019, https://www.healthline.com/nutrition/juicing-good-or-bad.

invested in a more practical one. If juicing is not your thing, make every effort to consume fruits and vegetables in their raw form to take full advantage of the nutrients.

There are some variables that you need to consider when consuming fruits and vegetables. Although all of them contain a variety of nutrients, some may not be easily absorbed by your body. This may be true for cruciferous vegetables like broccoli, cauliflower, and cabbage. These vegetables are high in sulfur. Foods high in sulfur get broken down in the large intestine and produce gas. This could be of particular concern for those suffering from irritable bowel syndrome, so consult your healthcare providers if you need further clarification or specific recommendations on particular fruits and vegetables that are best suited for you.

In his extraordinary book *The 9 Steps to Keep the Doctor Away*, Dr. Rashid A. Buttar stresses the importance of eating organic fruits and vegetables. He writes:

Invest in your health. We could go through virtually every existing fruit and vegetable, making these comparisons, but the results would be very much the same and equally dramatic.

The bottom line is that the foundation of all healing begins with what you put in your mouth. It's not enough to stop eating the pastries and candy bars. It's vital that you now begin to give your body the building blocks it needs for repair and regeneration. As you've just seen, an apple is not 'just' an apple. You must begin consuming more organic fruits and vegetables every day. Yes, organic produce can cost more, but consider this an investment in your own health that will pay dividends FAR beyond the few extra pennies you will spend.[58]

---

58   *The 9 Steps to Keep the Doctor Away*, p. 72.

CHAPTER 9

My "Easy Steps" to Regaining Wellness

I had a hard decision to make when I was diagnosed with cancer. My life was on the line, and I couldn't blindly surrender to a treatment that I knew was not going to benefit my general health and well-being. Getting healthier with alternative, holistic, natural approaches made more sense than utilizing a toxic medication.

The fact is that the majority of cancer cases are attributed to external factors rather than to genetic defects. I had to look to epigenetics for a sound solution. According to the *Journal of the American Association of Pharmaceutical Scientists*, "Only 5–10% of all cancer cases can be attributed to genetic defects, whereas the remaining 90–95% have their roots in the environment and lifestyle…Cancer continues to be a worldwide killer, despite the enormous amount of research and rapid developments seen during the past decade. According to recent statistics, cancer accounts for about 23% of the total deaths in the USA and is the second most common cause of death after heart disease."[59]

This data is cited by multiple reputable sources, including American Cancer Society, the National Library of Medicine, and the Cancer Support Community.

Amazingly, this means that most cancer can be prevented and even reversed if environmental and lifestyle factors are changed.[60]

Everything that I'll describe below worked for me, and I didn't experience any drawbacks, but as with any other disease, there is no one-size-fits-all solution. Rather, it is a combination of different approaches that we need to utilize to help our body and mind to heal.

Most of the practices I utilized are easy, practical to implement, inexpensive, and will help you immensely. Most of the recommendations, such as drinking sufficient water, deep breathing, exercising, getting enough sleep, and controlling your stress levels are common sense, though, unfortunately, they are not common practices. Understanding these easy steps for keeping my body in balance was pivotal to regaining my wellness.

WATER

An easy task such as drinking enough clean water is critical to keeping your body hydrated and your mind at ease. The benefits of drinking enough water during the day are enormous; however, if you are not used to doing it, you may struggle at the beginning.

One way to help you drink more water is to make it flavorful. Add some herbs or fruit or vegetable slices—strawberries, cucumber, mint, lemon—to a jug of water.

How much water is enough? Before I had cancer, I drank just one glass of water a day—way too little. Most experts recommend that women

59   Preetha Anand et al, "Cancer is a Preventable Disease that Requires Major Lifestyle Changes," *Pharmaceutical Research*, July 15, 2008, https://www.ncbi.nlm.nih.gov/pmc/articles/PMC2515569/.

60   "What Is Cancer?" National Cancer Institute, https://www.cancer.gov/about-cancer/understanding/what-is-cancer.

drink approximately 11.5 cups of fluid a day and men drink 15.5 cups daily.[61]

If you are not used to drinking that much water, start slowly, incorporating it until you reach your recommended amount. People who are used to drinking sugary drinks—I favored sweet carbonated beverages—may find it more of a challenge. Your palate might be so used to sweet drinks that to transition to water can be difficult. Remember that drinking enough liquids is not the same as drinking enough water.

Drinking water is probably the simplest but most important way to boost your lymphatic system. Similar to the waste plumbing in your home, your lymphatic system works more efficiently when it has water in it to move things along.

Dehydration is the primary cause of an underproductive lymphatic system. According to Harvard Medical School, water keeps *every* system in the body functioning properly. Water has many important jobs, such as:

- carrying nutrients and oxygen to the cells
- flushing bacteria from the bladder
- aiding digestion
- preventing constipation
- normalizing blood pressure
- stabilizing the heartbeat
- cushioning joints
- protecting organs and tissues
- regulating body temperature
- maintaining electrolyte (sodium) balance[62]

Warning signs of dehydration include weakness, low blood pressure,

---

61   "How much should you drink every day?" Mayo Clinic, accessed July 23, 2020, https://www.mayoclinic.org/healthy-lifestyle/nutrition-and-healthy-eating/in-depth/water/art-20044256.

62   "How much water should you drink?" Harvard Health Publishing, Harvard Medical School, updated March 25, 2020, https://www.health.harvard.edu/staying-healthy/how-much-water-should-you-drink.

dizziness, confusion, and urine that's dark in color. I remember getting lots of headaches, and I now attribute that to insufficient water consumption.

Fresh air impoverishes the doctor.

—DANISH PROVERB

DEEP BREATHING

Another important and free strategy for keeping your body in balance is oxygenating through proper breathing. Most people breath shallowly instead of breathing right from the stomach. You need to inhale through your nose, fill your lungs fully, and exhale completely to ensure you are doing deep belly breathing.

Sit comfortably, with your back straight. Put one hand on your chest and the other on your stomach. Breathe in through your nose. Exhale through your mouth, pushing out as much air as you can while contracting your abdominal muscles. Continue to breathe in through your nose and out through your mouth.

Five deep belly breaths disengage the stress response, which allows for optimal brain function, clear thoughts, and relaxation. You can practice this exercise several times during the day—while driving, lying down in bed, sitting, or standing. I set a phone alarm to remind me to intentionally practice proper breathing at least every hour. It won't take you more than a minute, but the results are substantial.

According a *New York Times* article, deep breathing appears to send signals to the brain to adjust the parasympathetic nervous system with multiple benefits. Some of the benefits of deep breathing include a reduction in stress and blood pressure, strengthening of abdominal and intestinal muscles, and relief of general body aches and pains.[63] Deep breathing

---

63   Lesley Alderman, "Breathe. Exhale, Repeat: The Benefits of Controlled Breathing," *New York Times*, November 9, 2019, https://www.nytimes.com/2016/11/09/well/mind/breathe-exhale-repeat-the-benefits-of-controlled-breathing.html.

also promotes better blood flow, releases toxins from the body, and aids in healthy sleep. Furthermore, deep breathing relaxes the mind and body and brings clarity and insights, thereby relieving emotional problems and clearing uneasy feelings from your body.

The movement of the diaphragm during deep breathing helps to massage your organs, primarily the stomach, small intestine, liver, pancreas, and heart. It strengthens the immune system so your body can better metabolize nutrients and vitamins. It helps to improve posture and assists with the digestion and assimilation of food.

It boosts energy and stamina, strengthens the heart and lungs, and nourishes the nervous system (brain, spinal cord, and nerves). Proper breathing even assists with weight control, as the extra oxygen helps burn up excess fat more efficiently. If you are underweight, it helps feed the starving glands and tissues.

REBOUNDING

My next-favorite activity is rebounding. Rebound exercise is a low-impact aerobic exercise often done on a "rebounder"—sometimes called a "mini trampoline"—which is three- or four-foot diameter version of a regular athletic trampoline. I learned about rebounding while researching alternative methods to treat cancer. I found out that it has enormous benefits, particularly in stimulating the lymphatic system. It gets drained through the skin during the rebounding activity.

Natural News reports that bouncing on a rebounder for two minutes every hour is good therapy for preventing or treating cancer. One hour after rebounding, the white blood cell count normalizes. Rebounding every hour will keep your immune system in optimum running condition.

I use the trampoline early in the morning before showering for about fifteen minutes. Bounce, dance, do jumping jacks (make sure you have proper clearance), run in place—any kind of vertical activity works. Plus, it's fun!

According to Cancer Tutor.com, the benefits of rebounding include:

- promoting lymphatic drainage and immune function;
- strengthening the skeletal system and increasing bone mass (it's twice as effective as running without putting extra stress on the ankles and knees);
- improving digestion;
- increasing endurance on a cellular level by stimulating mitochondrial production (which is responsible for cell energy);
- improving balance by stimulating the vestibule in the middle ear;
- Improving the effects of other exercises—one study found that those who rebounded for thirty seconds between weight lifting sets saw 25 percent more improvement after twelve weeks than those who did not;
- helping to circulate oxygen throughout the body and improving muscle tone.[64]

Certified lymphologists and reboundologists (yes, it is a real term) believe that vertical motion exercises such as rebounding are most effective for lymphatic actuation.

In *The Truth about Cancer*, Ty Bollinger writes, "A rebounder is basically a mini trampoline that, because of how it moves the body, is one of the most effective ways to optimize the lymphatic system.

"Making up about twenty-five percent of white blood cell content, lymphocytes, the primary cells of the lymphatic system, draw out and eliminate abnormal body cells, including those that are cancerous. Unlike blood, which has constantly circulating and working to filter out toxins from your tissue and cells regardless of your levels of physical activity, your lymph system only functions when you are physically active."

Rebounders are available in sporting goods stores as well online for a wide range of prices. If you're unable to invest in a rebounder, skipping

64   "Rebounding: Science Behind the 7 Major Health of Rebound Exercise," CancerTutor. com, December 27, 2019, https://www.cancertutor.com/rebounding/.

rope and doing jumping jacks are also vertical movements, but they will place considerably more stress on your joints.

DRY BRUSHING

My next free and favorite activity is dry brushing. As many of you know, our skin is the largest organ of absorption and elimination. Many people exfoliate the skin on their faces regularly, but the truth is that your whole body could do with thorough and regular exfoliation. Skin that is clogged with toxins and dead cells cannot function properly because the toxins are not being eliminated—and it is estimated that the skin eliminates over one pound of waste per day.

According to the Cleveland Clinic, dry brushing has several benefits, including boosting circulation, improving and firming the skin, unclogging pores, and invigorating the nervous system. In addition, it could help you feel more energetic, and it is said to help reduce cellulite.[65]

You can dry skin brush daily but do it a minimum of three times a week (and preferably five) for best results. A natural-bristled brush is best. Avoid nylon and synthetic brushes because they can scratch and irritate your skin. Brushes can be purchased in any drugstore or online. Get one with a long, detachable handle and a strip of cloth attached to the back of the brush for inserting your hand for a better grip.

COCONUT OIL PULLING

Coconut oil pulling is another superlow-cost practice. It helps to keep the mouth free from harmful bacteria that could lead to illness. It's an ancient Ayurvedic practice dating back more than three thousand years in which you swish a spoonful of extra virgin organic cold-pressed oil around in your mouth for twenty minutes on an empty stomach. (I use

---

65   Jamie Starkey, "The Truth about Dry Brushing and What It Does for You," Cleveland Clinic, January 26, 2015, https://health.clevelandclinic.org/the-truth-about-dry-brushing-and-what-it-does-for-you/.

coconut oil, but sesame or olive oil are fine, too.) Pull it between your teeth before spitting it out into the trash bin.

Do not spit it into your sink or toilet, as it may solidify and clog the pipes. Whatever you do, do not swallow the oil, as you will ingest the toxins you are trying to get rid of. Afterward, brush with fluoride-free toothpaste and rinse your mouth out. And you're done! It really is that easy.

Oil pulling can really transform your health. With the mouth as the home to millions of bacteria, fungi, viruses, and other toxins, the oil acts as a cleanser, pulling out nasties before they get a chance to spread throughout the body. This frees up the immune system, reduces stress, curtails internal inflammation, and aids well-being.[66]

Pure coconut oil is rich in lauric acid, a fatty acid also found in human breast milk. Lauric acid is beneficial in deterring parasites, bacteria, fungi, yeasts, and viruses.

Raw, organic, virgin coconut oil is considered a superfood because it helps among others to increase cardiovascular function, heals damaged cells that can lead to cancer and other diseases, and cleanses the body.[67]

THE BUDWIG PROTOCOL

The Budwig Protocol consists of eating organic flaxseed oil combined with organic, low-fat cottage cheese. According to the late Dr. Johanna Budwig, it has proven to cure many illnesses including cancer. In her book *Flax Oil as a True Aid Against Arthritis, Heart Infarction, Cancer and Other Diseases*, she writes, "Various highly trained and educated individuals are dismayed and irritated by the fact that serious medical conditions

---

66   J. Colquhoun, "The 7 Health Benefits of Oil Pulling," Food Matters, September 17, 2014, https://www. foodmatters.com/article/the-7-health-benefits-of-oil-pulling.

67   Bruce Fife, *The Coconut Oil Miracle*, fifth edition (New York: Penguin Random House, 2013) p. 4

can be cured by cottage cheese and flax seed oil."[68]

Dr. Johanna Budwig was born in Germany in 1908 and passed away in 2003 at the age of ninety-five. She was a top European cancer research scientist, biochemist, blood specialist, pharmacologist, and physicist. Dr. Budwig was a seven-time Nobel Prize nominee. She did not believe in the use of growth-inhibiting treatments such as chemotherapy or radiation. "I flat declare that the usual hospital treatments today, in a case of tumorous growth, most certainly leads to worsening of the disease or a speedier death, and in healthy people, quickly causes cancer," she said.[69] She was not the only doctor who truly believed that cancer can be healed in a less aggressive manner than with chemotherapy, and I was convinced of this early enough to refuse that treatment.

Dr. Budwig discovered that when she combined flaxseed oil, which contains essential electron-rich unsaturated fats with powerful healing properties, and cottage cheese, which is rich in sulfur protein, the chemical reaction that is produced makes the oil water soluble and easily absorbed by cell membranes. Simply put, the purpose of the Budwig Protocol (mixture of cold pressed organic flaxseed oil with cottage cheese) is to oxygenate the cells; healthy cells love oxygen—unlike cancer cells, which are anaerobic and die when they receive oxygen.[70]

There are various ways to prepare the Budwig recipe, but this is how I did it. I mixed three tablespoons of flaxseed oil and six tablespoons of cottage cheese and thoroughly blended the mixture until no oil showed. The two foods must be completely emulsified; you can add fresh fruit, fruit juice, raw nuts, or other flavorings. I usually used fresh pineapple to flavor it, and I drank this recipe every day, first thing in the morning.

---

68   Dr. Johanna Budwig, *Flax Oil as a True Aid Against Arthritis, Heart Infarction, Cancer and Other Diseases,* (Apple Publishing, 1994), p. 11.

69   Ursula Escher and Gene Wei, *A Day in the Budwig Diet,* (Scotts Valley, California: CreateSpace Independent Publishing Platform, 2011), p. 10.

70   *Beating Cancer with Nutrition,* p. 12.

THE HOXSEY METHOD

Concurrently with the Budwig Protocol, I used the Hoxsey tonic prescribed at the Bio Medical Center in Tijuana, Mexico. The Hoxsey Method is not new. Hoxsey clinics successfully operated in the United States during the 1950s and 1960s, documenting many cases of cured cancer, until the government shut them down in reaction to the allegation that it was quackery. That event forced the founder, Harry Hoxsey, to open new clinics in Mexico. The headquarters is in Tijuana, just across the border from San Diego.[71] The Hoxsey tonic consists a special formula prescribed by medical doctors at the clinic. Along with this protocol, a special diet should be followed, particularly during the treatment period.

Treatments available at the biomedical center also include natural herbs, special diets, vitamins and minerals, lifestyle counseling to maintain a positive attitude, and conventional medical treatments, when indicated. Modern diagnostic methods include extensive laboratory analysis, X-rays, ultrasound, and CT scans, as needed. Once an accurate diagnosis has been made, the doctors will outline a special program that works to strengthen the impaired immune system. By rebalancing and normalizing your metabolism, the treatments at the Bio Medical Center give your body a chance to heal itself, often without resorting to more toxic debilitating treatments.

During my visits to the Bio Medical Center, I had the opportunity to talk to patients who told me that they had gone to the clinic as a last resort because there was nothing more their doctors could do for them. Many of these people were now cancer free, and some had been cancer free for decades since their diagnoses.

You can read the testimonials of former and current patients on the Bio Medical Center's website.[72]

---

71   *The Truth about Cancer,* p. 41.

72   "Patient Testimonials," Hoxsey, accessed July 23, 2020, https://www.hoxseybiomedical. com/patient-testimonials/

HYPERBARIC OXYGEN THERAPY

In addition to the Budwig and Hoxsey protocols, I received thirty-five sessions of hyperbaric oxygen treatment. Hyperbaric oxygen therapy involves breathing pure oxygen in a pressurized room or tube.[73] Although this could be a pretty expensive treatment to pay for out of pocket, there are clinics and doctors in Mexico that charge about one hundred dollars per one-hour session.

In a hyperbaric oxygen therapy chamber, the air pressure is increased to three times higher than normal air pressure. Under these conditions, your lungs can gather more oxygen than would be possible breathing pure oxygen at normal air pressure. Your blood carries this oxygen throughout your body. This helps fight bacteria and stimulate the release of substances called growth factors and stem cells that promote healing.

This treatment accelerated my body's healing after going through the stress of radiation and surgery. I have to confess that I felt uneasy being inside the chamber for ninety minutes, but I always made a point of approaching it with hope and positivism.

> Physical fitness is not only one of the most important keys to a healthy body, it is the basis of dynamic and creative intellectual activity.
>
> —JOHN F. KENNEDY

EXERCISE

It's now general knowledge that exercise confers abundant benefits, particularly for health. During my recovery, I incorporated more consistent exercise into my regime. I am not an athlete, not even close. "Formal"

---

73   "Hyperbaric Oxygen Therapy," Mayo Clinic, https://www.mayoclinic.org/tests-procedures/ hyperbaric-oxygen-therapy/about/pac-20394380.

going-to-the-gym exercising is not my habit. I like walking and jogging; I like to ride a bike and jump on the minitrampoline, and that's what I did. The best thing about exercising is that adding it to your daily routine is easy if you take it slowly.

Initially, focus on small steps toward making your life more dynamic and active. For example, use the stairs as much as you can or park far from your location and jog the rest of the way. I bought a minitrampoline and started a bouncing regimen of up to twenty minutes daily. (This is "rebounding," described above.) Biking and walking were also part of my ongoing routine. It is essential that you check with your doctor first before you start any of these exercise programs.

Research shows that exercising lowers your risk for two types of cancer: colon and breast. Although the research is not yet final, it suggests that the risk of endometrial cancer and lung cancer may also be lower if you get regular physical activity.

If you are a cancer survivor, research shows that regular physical activity not only improves your physical fitness but also gives you a better quality of life.

In *The 9 Steps to Keep the Doctor Away*, Dr. Rashid A. Buttar writes, "Exercise dramatically elevates hormonal levels that govern every process and function in your body…exercise regulates your heart rate to a lower resting level, allowing the heart to function at a better pace. Stress-relieving endorphins are released, putting you in a better psychological space in which healing can occur. And lymphatic is stimulated, alleviating stagnation of the one system that is crucial-yet ignored by clinical medicine –in the prevention of chronic disease."

Exercising increases your chances of living longer. Science has shown that physical activity can reduce your risk of dying early from the leading causes of death, like heart disease and some cancers. This is remarkable because only a few "better-lifestyle" choices have as significant an impact on your wellness as physical activity. People who do moderate-intensity aerobic activity for about seven hours a week (an hour a day) have a lower risk of dying early than those who are active for less than thirty minutes a week. In his book *How Not to Die,* Dr. Greger writes, "And an hour-long walk each day may reduce mortality by 24 percent."[74]

The trouble with always trying to preserve the health of the body is that it is so difficult to do without destroying the health of the mind.

—G. K. CHESTERTON

PROTECT YOUR EMOTIONAL STATE

Stress is negative emotions like fear, anger, bitterness, resentment, unforgiveness, jealousy, envy, shame (being ashamed yourself or of your mistakes), regret, and anxiety. Basically, any negative emotion that you experience causes stress in your mind first, and then that stress manifests in physical ailments.

It is important that you not hold a grudge against anybody, for example. Try to remember that the other person is not suffering from your grudge; the only individual who will pay the consequences of unforgiveness in your heart is you. Try to banish those negative feelings to keep your mind at peace.

Your body is intelligently designed to save your life, assuming you know how to manage negative emotions. There are many programs for stress release available. I do not have a particular recommendation, but I followed a couple of techniques, such as simple meditation; practicing deep breathing, which I found very relaxing; listening to relaxing music; and exercising.

---

74   *How Not to Die,* p. 398.

> My own prescription for health is less paperwork and more
> running barefoot through the grass.
>
> —LESLIE GRIMUTTER

GROUNDING

Earthing (grounding) refers to the human body being in contact with the surface of the earth by barefoot exposure outdoors or by using special indoor systems connected to the earth. Studies have shown many beneficial effects of such contact include better sleep; normalization of cortisol; reduced inflammation, pain and stress; and better blood flow.[75]

The earth possesses a form of easily accessible, beneficial natural energy that has been demonstrated to influence human physiology and health positively. To determine if grounding for one hour improves facial blood circulation, forty middle-aged volunteers were divided into a grounded group and a sham-grounded group according to a double-blind procedure.

The results of this innovative study demonstrated, for the first time, that even one-hour contact with the surface of the earth appears to promote a significant increase in blood flow to the head and torso that may enhance skin tissue repair, health, and vitality, and optimize facial appearance.

Thermal imaging showed improved fluid movements in the abdomen as well as improved blood circulation to the face and throughout the torso, which in turn, may translate into better wellness. Further study, using larger comparison groups and a longer follow-up time, is warranted to confirm the influence of the earth as a protector of skin and overall

---

75   "One-Hour Contact with the Earth's Surface (Grounding) Improves Inflammation and Blood Flow—A Randomized, Double-Blind, Pilot Study," *Health*, Vol.7 No.8 (2015), DOI:10.4236/health.2015.78119.

health and well-being.[76]

DIETARY SUPPLEMENTS

The *Merriam-Webster* medical definition of a dietary supplement is, "A product taken orally that contains one or more ingredients (such as vitamins, minerals, herbs, or amino acids) that are intended to supplement one's diet and are not considered food."

In *Beating Cancer with Nutrition*, Dr. Patrick Quillin writes, "Cancer patients probably need more nutrients than can be obtained even from a healthy diet. No supplement is a magic bullet against cancer. Nutrition products need to be taken with professional guidance; the risk-to-ratio benefits heavily favor the use of supplements for all cancer patients. Supplements can stimulate immune function, encourage 'suicide' (apoptosis) in cancer cells, improve cell-to-cell communication and reduce the toxicity of chemo and radiation on the patient."

According to Dr. Quillen, there are now over twenty thousand scientific references that support the use of supplementing a good diet with vitamins, minerals, herbs, fatty acids, glandular, probiotics, and food extracts.

I personally included the following supplements in my regime: vitamin A, C, B, C, E, Quercitin, Beta 1, 3 glucan, turmeric, CQ-10, probiotics, enzymes, zinc, selenium, and astragalus.

But don't decide to take dietary supplements to treat a health condition that you have diagnosed yourself without consulting a health-care provider. Don't take supplements in place of, or in combination with, prescribed medications without your health-care provider's approval.

Check with your health-care provider about the supplements you take if you are scheduled to have any type of surgical procedure. The term *natural* doesn't always mean *safe*. A supplement's safety depends on many

---

76   "One-Hour Contact with the Earth's Surface (Grounding) Improves Inflammation and Blood Flow—A Randomized, Double-Blind, Pilot Study."

things, such as its chemical makeup, how it works in the body, how it is prepared, and the dose used. Certain herbs (for example, comfrey and kava) can harm the liver.[77]

REFLEXOLOGY

Reflexology, also known as zone therapy, is an ancient, alternative medicine involving the application of pressure to the feet and hands with specific thumb, finger, and hand techniques without the use of oil or lotion. Reflexology promotes a state of well-being and is a healing modality that has been practiced for two thousand years.

The benefits of reflexology include relieving back pain, chronic widespread pain and tenderness in the body, and migraines; helping with weight loss; and improving circulation and fibromyalgia. I am constantly looking for methods or approaches that will give my body what it needs, and I found reflexology to be very effective in helping me to relax. I saw improvement in my circulation, and even my digestive system improved.

My recommendation is to find a certified reflexologist with at least a year of experience. I began with weekly sessions for a period of two months, then went semiweekly, and finally, once a month.

If your resources are limited or reflexology is not within your reach, you could learn some basics of reflexology and try it on yourself. You could also partner with a family member or a friend and help each other.

AMETHYST PAD

During my journey of healing from cancer, I utilized every approach I came across that I considered to be sound and effective, including chiropractic, meditation, music therapy, prayer, reflexology, and energy healing through crystals.

There are several approaches to energy healing, and this modality has

---

77   "Strengthening Knowledge and Understanding of Dietary Supplements," National Institutes of Health, https://ods.od.nih.gov/HealthInformation/makingdecisions.sec.aspx.

gained popularity in recent years. However, energy healing is an ancient practice. I decided to buy an amethyst pad after watching a demonstration at a health conference I attended in San Diego, California.

Essentially, amethyst helps in the healing process when its naturally occurring magnetic field interacts with the human body's own magnetic field. In addition, the stone absorbs and reflects far infrared radiation, known to have an array of health benefits, such as supporting healthy cell growth. [78]

According to the amethyst literature, amethyst crystals helps to purify the blood, thus reducing physical, emotional, and psychological pain or stress. It is said to have antioxidant and bacteria-fighting properties and to boost cell regeneration and blood circulation. Amethyst is said to be useful for people suffering from diseases of the lungs and respiratory tract, skin conditions, disorders in cells, diseases of the digestive and immune systems, as well as for treatment of sleep disorders and addiction. Amethysts are also credited for helping with weight loss and rejuvenating the skin, thus delaying the aging process.[79]

HOW TO USE AMETHYST

The amethyst pad I used is similar to a yoga mat in size; however, it's heavier due to the many crystals it contains. The pad is plugged into a wall outlet to activate the crystals. Mine has a heat regulator so I can adjust the temperature. As per the manufacturer's instructions, it can be used daily. I lay on it for thirty minutes two or three times a week, at a medium temperature setting during my core treatment phase. In my experience, the most evident results were feeling more relaxed, sleeping better, and pain reduction. I am convinced it also provides other, less evident short- and long-term benefits.

---

78   "Amethyst: Meaning, Healing Properties and Powers," My Crystals, accessed July 23, 2020, https://www.mycrystals.com/meaning/amethyst-meaning-and-healing-properties.

79   "Amethyst: Meaning, Healing Properties and Powers."

It is recommended that you drink plenty of water before and after using amethyst, as it seems the heat depletes liquids in your body.

In her book *Heal Breast Cancer Naturally*, amethyst BioMat proponent Dr. Desaulniers cites National Cancer Institute data crediting high-temperature treatment for damaging and killing cancer cells.[80]

As always, consult with your health-care practitioner beforehand as Bio Mat could be contraindicated for people suffering with some chronic illnesses.

* * *

I believe this is a very important chapter of the book. It includes most of the strategies I used on my journey to regain wellness after going through cancer and recuperating from the side effects of surgery and radiation. I believe these strategies allowed me to become cancer free without chemotherapy.

These strategies will help most people tremendously regardless of their current health condition. If your health condition is good, they will help you to maintain and even improve it. If your health condition is not good, they will help you to get better.

Make a commitment today to act. If you're anything like me—somewhat resistant to change—go ahead and start slowly. It is better to start with baby steps and then increase them than it is to hit the road running and then quit.

---

80   *Heal Breast Cancer Naturally*, pp. 214-215.

CHAPTER 10

My Personal Recommendations

Carefully watch your thoughts, for they become your words. Manage and watch your words, for they will become your actions. Consider and judge your actions, for they have become your habits. Acknowledge and watch your habits, for they shall become your values. Understand and embrace your values, for they become your destiny.

—Mahatma Gandhi

I couldn't have selected a better quote than these words of Gandhi's to encourage you to take control of your life. If you don't, someone else will.

Our thoughts influence our words. Whatever occurs in our brain is what we usually talk about. If we articulate our thoughts, then most likely we will believe them. This means that your destiny is in your own hands. Your wellness is in your own hands. Your happiness is in your own hands and not in anyone else's—unless you allow it to be

My recommendations are straightforward. First, make sure that you are under the care of a licensed health-care professional who genuinely believes in the healing power of the human body. It could take some time to find one, but it is possible, as there are many of them.

Although the internet provides tons of information about health-care practitioners, make sure you consult trusted sites only. Word of mouth is one of the best ways to find them. Look for good reviews, but make sure you do your homework and investigate the doctors before placing your health in their hands. It is ultimately your responsibility to know who you are trusting with your wellness.

It typically takes just one visit to know if doctors care about your health. You can tell by the amount of time they spend with you and the number and quality of questions they ask.

Go to your appointments well prepared. Write down the questions you need to ask your doctor and write down the answers. Listen to other patients' recommendations and opinions. These are valuable to consider when selecting a *good* doctor.

If you are in doubt, leave and find another doctor. In the long run, you will save time by starting again. It will give you peace of mind to know that your health is in good hands.

Become aware of how cancer begins and flourishes in the human body. Cancer is not an isolated entity. For cancer to develop, healthy cells must become abnormal and multiply rapidly.

Since most cancers are diagnosed three to six years after they begin, know that you have time to consider options after your cancer is diagnosed. You do not have to rush into standard cancer treatment. You can use a reasonable amount of time to educate yourself on your type of cancer, its stage of development, the survival rate, and treatment options and their success rates. Treatment decisions are life-changing. Get educated on alternative, holistic, natural treatment options as well.

I'm happy with where I am now. However, I had to learn my lessons the hard way. I wish I had known in 2013 when my colon cancer was diagnosed what I know today. It would have saved me some struggles. I am convinced that I would not have gone through radiation and probably would not have undergone surgery. Had I been better educated about the risks and low effectiveness of standard cancer treatment, I might not have lost a kidney, because I would have been more aware of what my body was telling me and could have taken action earlier, when my kidney could have been saved. I wouldn't have gone through the stress and struggle of having the ileostomy.

These struggles made me realize how important it is to question doctors' orders. You need to place all facts in perspective and balance the pros and cons of every treatment. Prescribed medications sometimes produce more adverse side effects than the good they do for your body. Have you heard television commercials advertising medications for conditions such as diabetes and then mentioning a long list of adverse side effects?

Even simple over-the-counter medication can cause damage if taken for long periods of time. It is your responsibility to have a good understanding of what are you putting into your body. Make educated choices and do not allow others to rush you into a treatment regimen you are not comfortable with. Become aware, get educated, and take action.

Luckily, we are living in an era of rapid technological growth. All you need to do is access the internet, and the information pours in. Just make sure the sources are reputable.

Keep in mind that I am not telling you what to do. All I recommend is that you get educated using the available resources and, if necessary, have somebody help you. If you are reading this book and have a friend or relative going through a chronic health condition such as cancer, please understand that it is very important for patients to have someone they trust to mentor them and help them find alternative ways to treat their condition.

Your treatment is ultimately your choice to make. You can conquer cancer and continue living a wonderful life, full of hope and opportunities.

I believe that we are often given second and third opportunities in life. I believe that God was giving me a second chance through cancer. I am here in one piece, and it is my humble desire that this book will inspire you to educate yourself about your options for regaining wellness instead of blindly following doctors' orders.

I will close this chapter with a quote that motivates me and underscores the reason I wrote this book:

> If you're not making someone else's life better, then you are wasting your time. Your life will become better by making other people's lives better.
>
> —WILL SMITH

CHAPTER 11

RECOMMENDED RESOURCES

The books that I read at the beginning of my journey were *Beating Cancer with Nutrition* by Dr. Patrick Quillin and *Cancer-Free* by Bill Henderson. I later discovered and bought a docuseries called *The Quest for the Cures* by Ty Bollinger and a book by the same author called *The Truth About Cancer*, which includes interviews with several doctors along with testimonials from patients, as well as research conducted by Ty Bollinger.

Another interesting read is a book by Dr. Véronique Desaulniers, *Heal Breast Cancer Naturally*. I also followed some of the recommendations in the following books: *How Not to Die* by Dr. Michael Greger; *The 9 Steps to Keep the Doctor Away* by Dr. Rashid A. Buttar; *The China Study* by T. Collin Campbell, PhD, and Thomas M. Campbell II, MD; *One Man Alone* by Nicholas J. Gonzalez, MD; *The Naked Brain* by Richard Testak, MD; *Threshold of the Mind* by Bill Harris; *The Secret Food Cures* by Joan Wilen and Lydia Wilen; *The Deepest Well* by Nadine Burke Harris, MD; and *Your Erroneous Zones* by Wayne W. Dyer. These are just some of the resources that I delved into to research cancer and the body's healing mechanisms, and I highly recommend them.

I attended a health conference in San Diego, California in the spring of 2015, during which I heard many exceptional speakers, such as Dr. Antonio Jimenez, founder and medical director of the Hope4Cancer treatment centers in Mexico, and Dr. Francisco Contreras, director of Oasis of Hope Hospital in Tijuana, Mexico. I also learned about the Northern Baja Gerson Center in Rosarito, Baja, Mexico, and many medical institutions where alternative therapies are provided.

BIBLIOGRAPHY

Anand, P. et al. "Cancer is a Preventable Disease that Requires Major Lifestyle Changes." *Pharmaceutical Research*, July 15, 2008. https://www.ncbi.nlm.nih.gov/pmc/articles/PMC2515569/.

"Benefits of Physical Activity." Centers for Disease Control and Prevention. Accessed June 20, 2020. https://www.cdc.gov/physicalactivity/basics/pa-health/index.htm.

Bernstein, L. "Mom was right: Eat LOTS of veggies. (They're even better for you than fruit)." *The Washington Post*, April 1, 2014. Accessed June 20, 2020. https://www.washingtonpost.com/news/to-your-health/wp/2014/04/01/mom-was-right-eat-lots-of-veggies-theyre-even-better-for-you-than-fruit/.

Bollinger, Ty. *The Truth About Cancer*. Carlsbad, California: Hay House, 2018.

Budwig, Johanna. *Flax Oil as a True Aid Against Arthritis, Heart Infarction, Cancer and Other Diseases*. Apple Publishing, 1994.

Buttar, Rashid. *The 9 Steps to Keep the Doctor Away*. Lake Tahoe, Nevada: GMEC Publishing, 2010.

Campbell, Colin T., and Thomas Campbell, MD. *The China Study*. Dallas: BenBella Books, 2016.

"Cancer Epigenetics." Cancer Quest. Accessed October 14, 2018. https://www.cancerquest.org/cancer-biology/cancer-epigenetics.

"Cancer Statistics." National Cancer Institute. Accessed April 27, 2018. https://www.cancer.gov/ about-cancer/understanding/statistics.

Colquhoun, J. "The 7 Health Benefits of Oil Pulling." Food Matters (September 17, 2014). https://www.foodmatters.com/article/ the-7-health-benefits-of-oil-pulling.

Escher, Ursula and Gene Wei. *A Day in the Budwig Diet.* Scotts Valley, California: CreateSpace Independent Publishing Platform, 2011.

"EWG's Skin Deep." The Environmental Working Group.org. Accessed June 18, 2020. https://www.ewg.org/skindeep/.

Fife, Bruce, *The Coconut Oil Miracle*, fifth edition. New York: Penguin Random House, 2013.

Greger, Michael. *How Not to Die.* London: Pan MacMillan, 2015.

Group, E. "8 Benefits of Amethyst Gemstone," Global Healing. com. Updated February 22, 2017. https://globalhealing.com/ natural-health/8-benefits-amethyst-gemstone/.

Gunnars, K. "20 Delicious High Protein Foods." Healthline (March 3, 2020). https://www.healthline.com/nutrition/20-delicious-high-protein-foods.

"How Cancers Grow." Cancer Research UK. Accessed December 5, 2017. https://www.cancerresearchuk.org/about-cancer/what-is-cancer/ how-cancers-grow.

"How much water should you drink?" Harvard Health Publishing. Harvard Medical School. Updated March 25, 2020. https://www.health. harvard.edu/staying-healthy/how-much-water-should-you-drink.

"Hyperbaric Oxygen Therapy." Mayo Clinic. Accessed June 20, 2020. https:// www.mayoclinic.org/tests-procedures/hyperbaric-oxygen-therapy/ about/pac-20394380.

Liu, K. "Continuing to Fight; Nixon's War on Cancer." Richard Nixon Foundation. July 31, 2013. https://www.nixonfoundation.org/2013/07/continuing-to-fight-nixons-war-on-cancer/.

"One-Hour Contact with the Earth's Surface (Grounding) Improves Inflammation and Blood Flow—A Randomized, Double-Blind, Pilot Study." *Health*. Vol.7 No.8(2015). Paper ID 58836. 38 pages. DOI: 10.4236/health.2015.78119.

Quillin, Patrick. *Beating Cancer with Nutrition*. Carlsbad, California: Nutrition Times Press, 2005.

"Rebounding: Science Behind the 7 Major Benefits of Rebound Exercise." Cancer Tutor. Updated December 27, 2019. https://www.cancertutor.com/rebounding/.

Rudrappa, U. Nutrition Facts Blog. Accessed October 14, 2018. https://www. nutrition-and-you.com/.

Segerstrom, Suzanne C, and Gregory E. Miller. "Psychological stress and the human immune system: a meta-analytic study of 30 years of inquiry." *Psychological Bulletin* vol. 130,4 (2004): 601-30. doi:10.1037/0033-2909.130.4.601.

"Stomach Cancer Survival Rates." American Cancer Society. Accessed December 8, 2017. https:// www.cancer.org/cancer/stomach-cancer/detection-diagnosis-staging/survival-rates.html.

"Strengthening Knowledge and Understanding of Dietary Supplements." National Institutes of Health. Accessed June 20, 2020. https://ods.od.nih.gov/HealthInformation/makingdecisions.sec.aspx.

"Taking care of yourself with Cologuard." Cologuard. Accessed June 20, 2020. https://www.cologuardtest.com/meet-cologuard.

The Truth About Cancer.com. Accessed October 14, 2018. https://thetruthaboutcancer.com/.

Urschel, Harold III. *Healing the Addicted Brain: The Revolutionary Science-Based Alcoholism and Addiction Recovery Program.* Naperville, Illinois: Sourcebooks, 2009.

Weil, Andrew. "Budwig Cure for Cancer?" *Weil.* December 20, 2017. https://www.drweil.com/health-wellness/ body-mind-spirit/cancer/ budwig-cure-for-cancer/.

Wells, K. "Health Benefits of Rebounding." Wellness Mama. Revised May 22, 2020. https://wellnessmama.com/13915/ rebounding-benefits/.

"What Is Cancer?" American Cancer Society. Accessed June 18, 2020. https://www.cancer.org/cancer/cancer-basics/what-is-cancer.html.

"What is Cancer?" Cancer Institute NSW. Accessed June 28, 2018. https:/ www.cancerinstitute.org.au/ understanding-cancer/what-is-cancer.

"What is cancer?" Cancer Treatment Centers of America. Accessed June 18, 2020. https://www.cancercenter.com/what-is-cancer.

"What Is Cancer?" National Cancer Institute, Accessed June 18, 2020. https://www.cancer.gov/about-cancer/understanding/what-is-cancer.

"What is BPA?" Mayo Clinic. Accessed March 11, 2016. https://www.mayoclinic.org/healthy- lifestyle/nutrition-and-healthy-eating/ expert-answers/bpa/ faq-20058331.

"What is Integrative Medicine?" WebMD. Updated May 25, 2019. https://www.webmd.com/cancer/holistic-treatment-17/ integrative-medicine.

"What Is Holistic Medicine?" WebMD. Updated March 18, 2020. https:// www.webmd.com/balance/guide/ what-is-holistic-medicine#1